BUSINESS AND GENERAL REFERENCE BOOK SERIES FROM IDG

Stephanie Seymour's
Beauty Secrets For Dumm

D0517573

Keeping Your Skin at Its Best

Use these tips to keep your skin looking great all the time:

✔ Drink plenty of water, eat a healthy diet, exercise, keep stress to a minimum, get enough sleep, and don't smoke.

✔ Never go straight to bed without taking care of your skin, even if you're exhausted. At the very least, wash your face with your cleanser.

✔ When you've used heavy makeup, cleanse your face with a makeup remover and then your cleanser, twice if necessary.

✔ If you use products containing AHAs or tretinoin, which can be very drying, make sure to use a moisturizer.

✔ Gently exfoliate your skin regularly to keep it smooth and give it a healthy glow. Regular exfoliation also allows your skin to absorb moisturizer better and helps makeup cover more smoothly.

✔ Use eye creams and gels to help reduce puffiness and improve the appearance of dark undereye circles.

✔ Always use a facial sunscreen with an SPF of 30 or higher.

Finding Your Style

No single makeup look or hairstyle looks right on every woman. And you shouldn't have just one look that you wear every day, either. To find a look that works for you or a new look for a special occasion, consider the following factors:

✔ Your age

✔ Your lifestyle

✔ Your mood

✔ Your personality

✔ Your destination

✔ The weather

✔ The season

✔ The time of day

✔ Your skin condition

✔ Changes in your coloring

✔ Your hairstyling and makeup application skills

Checking Your Makeup

After you complete all your makeup steps, take one last look. Here's a checklist of common slip-ups to look for:

✔ Make sure that you see no line of demarcation between your face and neck.

✔ Check your eyebrows and hair for residual foundation or powder.

✔ Dust off any excess powder.

✔ Remove any concealer that may have ended up on your lower lashes during application.

✔ Make sure that your blush is not streaking or applied too heavily.

✔ Remove any eye shadow sprinkles under the eyes or on the cheeks.

✔ Check your lipstick shape up close in a mirror or in a magnifying mirror, and smile to check for lipstick on the teeth.

...For Dummies: Bestselling Book Series for Beginners

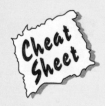

Cheat Sheet

BUSINESS AND
GENERAL
REFERENCE
BOOK SERIES
FROM IDG

Fixing Makeup Mistakes

Whether your hand slipped or you got carried away, you can always find a way to fix a makeup mistake without going back to the drawing board:

✔ **Too-heavy foundation:** Spray your face with a very fine mist of water and blot with a tissue; blend with a damp makeup sponge; or dab a little moisturizer on your fingers and blend over your face.

✔ **Overpowdered face:** Whisk away excess powder with a powder brush; press powder into the face with a velvet puff; or lightly spray the face with a fine mist of water.

✔ **Cakey concealer:** Dab a little moisturizer onto the area and blend.

✔ **Overcolored eyebrows:** Brush in a little loose powder; or use a hard toothbrush lightly coated with a neutral eye shadow and comb through.

✔ **Too-dark eye shadow:** Blend loose powder over the lid.

✔ **Hard-looking eyeliner:** Cover the line with loose powder or a lighter-toned eye shadow; or blend over the area with a brush or sponge-tip applicator (dry or damp).

✔ **Clumpy eyelashes:** Use a lash comb to remove clumps.

✔ **Mascara smudge:** Dampen a cotton swab with water or non-oily eye makeup remover, press onto the smudge with a blotting or twisting motion, and spot-reapply makeup if necessary.

✔ **Too much blush:** Blend loose powder over blush; or use a cotton ball to pick up a bit of color.

✔ **Too-bright lipstick:** Blot and then blend on a deeper or more neutral shade.

✔ **Too-dark lipstick:** Blot and then top-coat with a lighter shade; or blot and use as a stain, putting lip gloss or lip balm on top to make it look moist and natural. You can also use a dot of foundation mixed with lip gloss to lighten the color.

✔ **Lopsided lipstick:** Clean up anything over the lip line with a sponge wedge or cotton swab (dipped in makeup remover if the color is dense). If needed, reapply foundation with the edge of a sponge; then redefine the lip border with a lip pencil or brush.

✔ **Too-dry lipstick:** Add a coat of lip balm or gloss.

More Praise for Stephanie Seymour's
Beauty Secrets For Dummies

"*Beauty Secrets For Dummies* offers insider tips from a world-class beauty; anyone can find useful information here."

—Elaine Irwin Mellencamp, Supermodel

"Stephanie gives her personal touch on how to apply makeup with a sense of style. Thorough, fun, and an easy approach to beauty basics."

—Kelly Klein

"You'd have to be a 'dummy' not to buy this book! After all, who else but Stephanie Seymour could tell you how to look like a supermodel after three babies?"

—Veronica Webb, Model and Author of *Veronica Webb's Sight:
Adventures in the Big City*

"At last, someone in the world of beauty and fashion has written a book with a no-nonsense approach to beauty and skin care. Stephanie Seymour makes beauty obtainable for all women. *Beauty Secrets For Dummies* provides everything I ever wanted to know about beauty but was afraid to ask."

—Annette Tapert, Author of *The Power of Glamour* and
Co-author of *The Power of Style*

"Stephanie Seymour is one of the most genuinely beautiful women I know. She has a purity and grace that shines through in all that she is — wife, mother, and supermodel."

—Elizabeth Saltzman, Fashion Director, *Vanity Fair* Magazine

Stephanie's beauty secrets on hair are an invaluable source of information. From finding your individual style and color to basic hair care, this book outlines everything in easy-to-follow steps. If you are one of the many women who suffer from a bad haircut or color, or would like to avoid these hair disasters, Stephanie's book is a must-have guide to beautiful hair.

—John Frieda

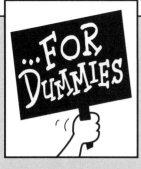 ™

References for the Rest of Us! ®

BESTSELLING BOOK SERIES FROM IDG

Are you intimidated and confused by computers? Do you find that traditional manuals are overloaded with technical details you'll never use? Do your friends and family always call you to fix simple problems on their PCs? Then the *...For Dummies*® computer book series from IDG Books Worldwide is for you.

...For Dummies books are written for those frustrated computer users who know they aren't really dumb but find that PC hardware, software, and indeed the unique vocabulary of computing make them feel helpless. *...For Dummies* books use a lighthearted approach, a down-to-earth style, and even cartoons and humorous icons to diffuse computer novices' fears and build their confidence. Lighthearted but not lightweight, these books are a perfect survival guide for anyone forced to use a computer.

Already, millions of satisfied readers agree. They have made *...For Dummies* books the #1 introductory level computer book series and have written asking for more. So, if you're looking for the most fun and easy way to learn about computers, look to *...For Dummies* books to give you a helping hand.

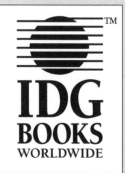
™

IDG BOOKS WORLDWIDE

8/98

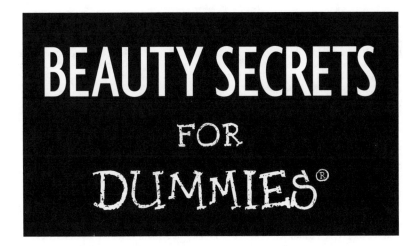

BEAUTY SECRETS FOR DUMMIES®

by Stephanie Seymour

Foreword by Sarah,
The Duchess of York

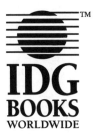

IDG Books Worldwide, Inc.
An International Data Group Company

Foster City, CA ♦ Chicago, IL ♦ Indianapolis, IN ♦ New York, NY

Beauty Secrets For Dummies®

Published by
IDG Books Worldwide, Inc.
An International Data Group Company
919 E. Hillsdale Blvd.
Suite 400
Foster City, CA 94404
www.idgbooks.com (IDG Books Worldwide Web site)
www.dummies.com (Dummies Press Web site)

Library of Congress Catalog Card No.: 98-87438

ISBN: 0-7645-5078-0

Printed in the United States of America

10 9 8 7 6 5 4 3 2 1

1E/RX/QZ/ZY/IN

Distributed in the United States by IDG Books Worldwide, Inc.

Distributed by Macmillan Canada for Canada; by Transworld Publishers Limited in the United Kingdom; by IDG Norge Books for Norway; by IDG Sweden Books for Sweden; by Woodslane Pty. Ltd. for Australia; by Woodslane (NZ) Ltd. for New Zealand; by Addison Wesley Longman Singapore Pte Ltd. for Singapore, Malaysia, Thailand, Indonesia and Korea; by Norma Comunicaciones S.A. for Colombia; by Intersoft for South Africa; by International Thomson Publishing for Germany, Austria and Switzerland; by Toppan Company Ltd. for Japan; by Distribuidora Cuspide for Argentina; by Livraria Cultura for Brazil; by Ediciencia S.A. for Ecuador; by Ediciones ZETA S.C.R. Ltda. for Peru; by WS Computer Publishing Corporation, Inc., for the Philippines; by Unalis Corporation for Taiwan; by Contemporanea de Ediciones for Venezuela; by Computer Book & Magazine Store for Puerto Rico; by Express Computer Distributors for the Caribbean and West Indies. Authorized Sales Agent: Anthony Rudkin Associates for the Middle East and North Africa.

For general information on IDG Books Worldwide's books in the U.S., please call our Consumer Customer Service department at 800-762-2974. For reseller information, including discounts and premium sales, please call our Reseller Customer Service department at 800-434-3422.

For information on where to purchase IDG Books Worldwide's books outside the U.S., please contact our International Sales department at 650-655-3200 or fax 650-655-3297.

For information on foreign language translations, please contact our Foreign & Subsidiary Rights department at 650-655-3021 or fax 650-655-3281.

For sales inquiries and special prices for bulk quantities, please contact our Sales department at 650-655-3200 or write to the address above.

For information on using IDG Books Worldwide's books in the classroom or for ordering examination copies, please contact our Educational Sales department at 800-434-2086 or fax 317-596-5499.

For press review copies, author interviews, or other publicity information, please contact our Public Relations department at 650-655-3000 or fax 650-655-3299.

For authorization to photocopy items for corporate, personal, or educational use, please contact Copyright Clearance Center, 222 Rosewood Drive, Danvers, MA 01923, or fax 978-750-4470.

About the Author

Stephanie Seymour is one of the fashion world's true supermodels. Since the age of 15, she has graced the covers of magazines all over the world, including *Allure, Cosmopolitan, Elle, Marie Claire, Vogue,* and *W.* She has been photographed by the most famous photographers of the last four decades. Richard Avedon calls her the single most interesting and powerful model he has ever photographed.

Stephanie is known as the face and figure of Victoria's Secret and has also acted as their spokesperson. She has done numerous campaigns for beauty and hair companies, such as Pantene, L'Oreal, and Almay, as well as many fashion campaigns, including Azzedine Alaia, Chanel, Ralph Lauren, Gianni Versace, and Yves Saint Laurent. Throughout her career as a model, Stephanie has learned her beauty tips from the best makeup artists, hairstylists, doctors, and beauty specialists.

Stephanie's first career is being a mother. Unique among professional models, she is the proud mother of three boys and is also very proud of her extended family from her marriage to Peter Brant, which includes five stepchildren.

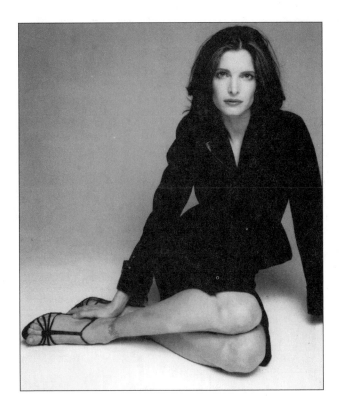

About the Photographer

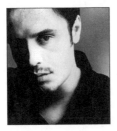

One of the most celebrated makeup artists in the world, **François Nars** (who designed and photographed the makeup looks for the color Makeup Workbook) is widely regarded as makeup's most influential modern talent. The dramatic, beautiful faces he designs for the runways of New York, Paris, and Milan become the blueprints for next season's definitive hot look.

Famed for his versatility and his imaginative and daring approach, François is at the pinnacle of his profession. His work is featured not only on the runways of designers like Versace, Valentino, Dolce and Gabbana, and Karl Lagerfeld, but also on the covers of magazines, including *Vogue, Harper's Bazaar, W, Allure,* and *Elle,* and in influential advertising campaigns for clients such as Calvin Klein and Ralph Lauren. Many famous faces, such as Madonna, Sharon Stone, Lauren Hutton, Michelle Pfeiffer, Isabella Rosselini, Anjelica Houston, and Catherine Deneuve, have benefited from his dynamic sense of color and finely honed technique. François's constant drive for perfection led him to begin developing his own line of cosmetics in 1994.

ABOUT IDG BOOKS WORLDWIDE

Welcome to the world of IDG Books Worldwide.

IDG Books Worldwide, Inc., is a subsidiary of International Data Group, the world's largest publisher of computer-related information and the leading global provider of information services on information technology. IDG was founded more than 25 years ago and now employs more than 8,500 people worldwide. IDG publishes more than 275 computer publications in over 75 countries (see listing below). More than 90 million people read one or more IDG publications each month.

Launched in 1990, IDG Books Worldwide is today the #1 publisher of best-selling computer books in the United States. We are proud to have received eight awards from the Computer Press Association in recognition of editorial excellence and three from *Computer Currents'* First Annual Readers' Choice Awards. Our best-selling *...For Dummies®* series has more than 50 million copies in print with translations in 38 languages. IDG Books Worldwide, through a joint venture with IDG's Hi-Tech Beijing, became the first U.S. publisher to publish a computer book in the People's Republic of China. In record time, IDG Books Worldwide has become the first choice for millions of readers around the world who want to learn how to better manage their businesses.

Our mission is simple: Every one of our books is designed to bring extra value and skill-building instructions to the reader. Our books are written by experts who understand and care about our readers. The knowledge base of our editorial staff comes from years of experience in publishing, education, and journalism — experience we use to produce books for the '90s. In short, we care about books, so we attract the best people. We devote special attention to details such as audience, interior design, use of icons, and illustrations. And because we use an efficient process of authoring, editing, and desktop publishing our books electronically, we can spend more time ensuring superior content and spend less time on the technicalities of making books.

You can count on our commitment to deliver high-quality books at competitive prices on topics you want to read about. At IDG Books Worldwide, we continue in the IDG tradition of delivering quality for more than 25 years. You'll find no better book on a subject than one from IDG Books Worldwide.

IDG BOOKS WORLDWIDE

John Kilcullen
CEO
IDG Books Worldwide, Inc.

Steven Berkowitz
President and Publisher
IDG Books Worldwide, Inc.

Eighth Annual Computer Press Awards ➣1992

Ninth Annual Computer Press Awards ➣1993

Tenth Annual Computer Press Awards ➣1994

Eleventh Annual Computer Press Awards ➣1995

IDG Books Worldwide, Inc., is a subsidiary of International Data Group, the world's largest publisher of computer-related information and the leading global provider of information services on information technology. International Data Group publishes over 275 computer publications in over 75 countries. More than 90 million people read one or more International Data Group publications each month. International Data Group's publications include: **ARGENTINA:** Buyer's Guide, Computerworld Argentina, PC World Argentina; **AUSTRALIA:** Australian Macworld, Australian PC World, Australian Reseller News, Computerworld, IT Casebook, Network World, Publish, Webmaster; **AUSTRIA:** Computerwelt Osterreich, Networks Austria, PC Tip Austria; **BANGLADESH:** PC World Bangladesh; **BELARUS:** PC World Belarus; **BELGIUM:** Data News; **BRAZIL:** Annuário de Informática, Computerworld, Connections, Macworld, PC Player, PC World, Publish, Reseller News, Supergamepower; **BULGARIA:** Computerworld Bulgaria, Network World Bulgaria, PC & MacWorld Bulgaria; **CANADA:** CIO Canada, Client/Server World, ComputerWorld Canada, InfoWorld Canada, NetworkWorld Canada, WebWorld; **CHILE:** Computerworld Chile, PC World Chile; **COLOMBIA:** Computerworld Colombia, PC World Colombia; **COSTA RICA:** PC World Centro America; **THE CZECH AND SLOVAK REPUBLICS:** Computerworld Czechoslovakia, Macworld Czech Republic, PC World Czechoslovakia; **DENMARK:** Communications World Danmark, Computerworld Danmark, Macworld Danmark, PC World Danmark, Techworld Denmark; **DOMINICAN REPUBLIC:** PC World Republica Dominicana; **ECUADOR:** PC World Ecuador; **EGYPT:** Computerworld Middle East, PC World Middle East; **EL SALVADOR:** PC World Centro America; **FINLAND:** MikroPC, Tietoverkko, Tietoviikko; **FRANCE:** Distributique, Hebdo, Info PC, Le Monde Informatique, Macworld, Reseaux & Telecoms, WebMaster France; **GERMANY:** Computer Partner, Computerwoche, Computerwoche Extra, Computerwoche FOCUS, Global Online, Macwelt, PC Welt; **GREECE:** Amiga Computing, GamePro Greece, Multimedia World; **GUATEMALA:** PC World Centro America; **HONDURAS:** PC World Centro America; **HONG KONG:** Computerworld Hong Kong, PC World Hong Kong, Publish in Asia; **HUNGARY:** ABCD CD-ROM, Computerworld Szamitastechnika, Internetto online Magazine, PC World Hungary, PC-X Magazin Hungary; **ICELAND:** Tolvuheimur PC World Island; **INDIA:** Information Communications World, Information Systems Computerworld, PC World India, Publish in Asia; **INDONESIA:** InfoKomputer PC World, Komputek Computerworld, Publish in Asia; **IRELAND:** ComputerScope, PC Live!; **ISRAEL:** Macworld Israel, People & Computers/Computerworld; **ITALY:** Computerworld Italia, Macworld Italia, Networking Italia, PC World Italia; **JAPAN:** DTP World, Macworld Japan, Nikkei Personal Computing, OS/2 World Japan, SunWorld Japan, Windows NT World, Windows World Japan; **KENYA:** PC World East African; **KOREA:** Hi-Tech Information, Macworld Korea, PC World Korea; **MACEDONIA:** PC World Macedonia; **MALAYSIA:** Computerworld Malaysia, PC World Malaysia, Publish in Asia; **MALTA:** PC World Malta; **MEXICO:** Computerworld Mexico, PC World Mexico; **MYANMAR:** PC World Myanmar; **NETHERLANDS:** Computer! Totaal, LAN Internetworking Magazine, LAN World Buyers Guide, Macworld Netherlands, Net, WebWereld; **NEW ZEALAND:** Absolute Beginners Guide and Plain & Simple Series, Computer Buyer, Computer Industry Directory, Computerworld New Zealand, MTB, Network World, PC World New Zealand; **NICARAGUA:** PC World Centro America; **NORWAY:** Computerworld Norge, CW Rapport, Datamagasinet, Financial Rapport, Kursguide Norge, Macworld Norge, Multimediaworld Norge, PC World Ekspress Norge, PC World Nettverk, PC World Norge, PC World ProduktGuide Norge; **PAKISTAN:** Computerworld Pakistan; **PANAMA:** PC World Panama; **PEOPLE'S REPUBLIC OF CHINA:** China Computer Users, China Computerworld, China InfoWorld, China Telecom World Weekly, Computer & Communication, Electronic Design China, Electronics Today, Electronics Weekly, Game Software, PC World China, Popular Computer Week, Software Weekly, Software World, Telecom World; **PERU:** Computerworld Peru, PC World Profesional Peru, PC World SoHo Peru; **PHILIPPINES:** Click!, Computerworld Philippines, PC World Philippines, Publish in Asia; **POLAND:** Computerworld Poland, Computerworld Special Report Poland, Cyber, Macworld Poland, Networld Poland, PC World Komputer; **PORTUGAL:** Cerebro/PC World, Computerworld/Correio Informático, Dealer World Portugal, Mac*In/PC*In Portugal, Multimedia World; **PUERTO RICO:** PC World Puerto Rico; **ROMANIA:** Computerworld Romania, PC World Romania, Telecom Romania; **RUSSIA:** Computerworld Russia, Mir PK, Publish, Seti; **SINGAPORE:** Computerworld Singapore, PC World Singapore, Publish in Asia; **SLOVENIA:** Monitor; **SOUTH AFRICA:** Computing SA, Network World SA, Software World SA; **SPAIN:** Communicaciones World España, Computerworld España, Dealer World España, Macworld España, PC World España; **SRI LANKA:** Infolink PC World; **SWEDEN:** CAP&Design, Computer Sweden, Corporate Computing Sweden, Internetworld Sweden, it.branschen, Macworld Sweden, MaxiData Sweden, MikroDatorn, Natverk & Kommunikation, PC World Sweden, PCAktiv, Windows World Sweden; **SWITZERLAND:** Computerworld Schweiz, Macworld Schweiz, PCtip; **TAIWAN:** Computerworld Taiwan, Macworld Taiwan, NEW ViSiON/Publish, PC World Taiwan, Windows World Taiwan; **THAILAND:** Publish in Asia, Thai Computerworld; **TURKEY:** Computerworld Turkiye, Macworld Turkiye, Network World Turkiye, PC World Turkiye; **UKRAINE:** Computerworld Kiev, Multimedia World Ukraine, Network World Ukraine, PC World Ukraine; **UNITED KINGDOM:** Acorn User UK, Amiga Action UK, Amiga Computing UK, Apple Talk UK, Computing, Macworld, Parents and Computers UK, PC Advisor, PC Home, PSX Pro, The WEB; **UNITED STATES:** Cable in the Classroom, CIO Magazine, Computerworld, DOS World, Federal Computer Week, GamePro Magazine, InfoWorld, I-Way, Macworld, Network World, PC Games, PC World, Publish, Video Event, THE WEB Magazine, and WebMaster; online webzines: JavaWorld, NetscapeWorld, and SunWorld Online; **URUGUAY:** InfoWorld Uruguay; **VENEZUELA:** Computerworld Venezuela, PC World Venezuela; and **VIETNAM:** PC World Vietnam.   5/7/98

Author's Acknowledgments

I would like to start by thanking my editors, Tami Booth and Pam Mourouzis, for their endless and uncompromising support. I would also like to thank my dear friends and expert contributors, without whom this book would not have been possible: Max Pinnell, Glenn Marziali, Fran Cooper, Patricia Wexler, M.D., Frederic Fekkai, Howard Fuglar, François Nars, Elisa Ferri, Joel Kassimir, M.D., Fred Brandt, M.D., Phillippe Barr, Kelly Bensimon, H. Michael Roarke, M.D. Thanks also go to Laurie James, who helped me organize my thoughts and develop a first draft of much of the manuscript.

The color section couldn't have come together without the expertise and talent of François Nars and his hair and makeup team. Thanks, too, to the models who generously donated their time: Margaret Seymour, Daniela Pestova, Carmen, Raquel, Margareth, Tatjana, Yamila, and Ling. I would also like to thank the photographers for their generosity in giving me some of my favorite images of myself to work with: Miles Aldridge, Gilles Bensimon, Pamela Hanson, Russell James, Herb Ritts, Antoine Verglas, Ellen von Unwerth, and especially Patrick Demarchelier for his continued generosity in contributing his talents and photography to my book.

Lastly, I'd like to dedicate this book to two people: my mother for teaching me that it's more than okay to take care of yourself; it's a necessity and an important part of being a woman, and my dear friend and brilliant makeup artist George Newell for teaching me the power of makeup and for being a trusted and wonderful friend. I miss you.

Publisher's Acknowledgments

We're proud of this book; please register your comments through our IDG Books Worldwide Online Registration Form located at http://my2cents.dummies.com.

Some of the people who helped bring this book to market include the following:

Acquisitions, Development, and Editorial

Senior Project Editor: Pamela Mourouzis

Executive Editor: Tammerly Booth

Copy Editor: Tamara Castleman

Editorial Manager: Colleen Rainsberger

Editorial Coordinator: Maureen F. Kelly

Acquisitions Coordinator: Karen S. Young

Special Help

Wendy Hatch, Copy Editor; Heather Prince, Research Coordinator; Allison Solomon, Administrative Assistant

Production

Project Coordinator: E. Shawn Aylsworth

Layout and Graphics: Lou Boudreau, Angela F. Hunckler, Drew R. Moore, Anna Rohrer, Brent Savage, Janet Seib, Deirdre Smith, Kate Snell

Special Art: Monika Kim

Stock Photography: Everett Collection, Inc.; Shooting Star

Color Section: François Nars, Photography; Greg Broom, Photography; Jennifer Waverek, Design and Layout

Proofreaders: Nancy Price, Nancy L. Reinhardt, Janet M. Withers

Indexer: Christine Spina

General and Administrative

IDG Books Worldwide, Inc.: John Kilcullen, CEO; Steven Berkowitz, President and Publisher

IDG Books Technology Publishing: Brenda McLaughlin, Senior Vice President and Group Publisher

Dummies Technology Press and Dummies Editorial: Diane Graves Steele, Vice President and Associate Publisher; Mary Bednarek, Director of Acquisitions and Product Development; Kristin A. Cocks, Editorial Director

Dummies Trade Press: Kathleen A. Welton, Vice President and Publisher; Kevin Thornton, Acquisitions Manager

IDG Books Production for Dummies Press: Michael R. Britton, Vice President of Production and Creative Services; Beth Jenkins Roberts, Production Director; Cindy L. Phipps, Manager of Project Coordination, Production Proofreading, and Indexing; Kathie S. Schutte, Supervisor of Page Layout; Shelley Lea, Supervisor of Graphics and Design; Debbie J. Gates, Production Systems Specialist; Robert Springer, Supervisor of Proofreading; Debbie Stailey, Special Projects Coordinator; Tony Augsburger, Supervisor of Reprints and Bluelines

Dummies Packaging and Book Design: Robin Seaman, Creative Director; Jocelyn Kelaita, Product Packaging Coordinator; Joel Avirom, Cover Design

♦

The publisher would like to give special thanks to Patrick J. McGovern, without whom this book would not have been possible.

♦

Contents at a Glance

Table of Contents

Foreword

· ·

*W*hen I was asked to write the foreword for Stephanie's book, I felt greatly honoured and privileged. To me, Stephanie is a wonderful example of great beauty, and I admire her radiance and inner grace.

To me, writing the foreword of a beauty book seems to be a little ironic, as I often delight in not having to put on my makeup and have my hair styled, as I feel most comfortable with my natural look. However, I do take great pleasure in being fit and dressing well. I have found a personal style that works well for me, and I am no longer reticent about letting it show.

My knowledge of cosmetics, hair, and skin care is somewhat limited. However, like many women, I have little time to try the latest beauty products and cosmetics, so having a friend like Stephanie, who has shared so many of her beauty tips with me, is an enormous benefit. When you read this book and discover the secrets of beauty, your life will become easier, as mine has.

I admire Stephanie's approach to beauty, which begins with a healthy lifestyle. I also respect the intelligent way in which Stephanie has researched and organized the material in this book, giving the reader the ultimate beauty manual that is complete with proven tips and techniques from the world's leading beauty experts. This book will appeal to women of all ages and backgrounds, of all appearances and attitudes toward beauty. Providing us with the right information, Stephanie has removed many obstacles and myths and shows us the way forward in looking and feeling our very best.

On a more personal note, I would like to thank Stephanie for help, guidance, and valuable advice, both to me and to my mother. She is, quite simply, one in a million.

—Sarah, The Duchess of York

Introduction

- -

*A*lthough you may envy the long, perfectly straight hair of the woman in the office next door, never forget that the grass is always greener on the other side: She probably wants your masses of curly locks. The most important thing that I always stress to women who ask my advice on beauty is that everyone has something that makes her unique and special and beautiful. You may have unusually perfect skin or incredibly beautiful eyes. Whatever your unique feature is, it's important to know what it is and to embrace it. You don't have to follow trends or look like anybody else. You just need to be you, feel comfortable being you, and find your own personal style that plays up your beautiful features. In this book, I give my personal tips for finding your own style to make your best assets shine through.

About This Book

You don't have to read this book straight through or cover to cover to get the most out of it. Use this book as a reference. Jump from skin to makeup to hair, depending on what you need. For example, you may want to use this book for ideas to change your look for a special occasion. Whatever your beauty question or query may be, the answers are here. This book is meant to be kept not in your library or on your coffee table, but in your bathroom, where you need it and will use it.

Who You Are

In order to give you the most thorough information available (and the greatest quantity), I'm making some assumptions about you, the reader:

- **You're nobody's fool.** You may be overwhelmed by all the advertising, product choices, and conflicting advice, but you're smart enough to look for the answers.

- **You're female.** Of course men are interested in looking great, but women are obsessed with it. I've written this book with the purpose of reaching out specifically to women.

✔ **You're looking for tips and tricks to solve basic beauty problems.** No matter whether you're looking for tips on makeup, hair care, skin care, or beauty maintenance, you need sound advice for real women that you can put to use.

Whether you're a young girl who's just starting to experiment with cosmetics and other beauty products or an older woman with years of experience, this book has the answers you need.

How This Book Is Organized

This book is divided into four parts, each dealing with a separate facet of all-over beauty.

✔ **Part I, "Skin Care":** This part explains how your skin works and what you can do to keep it looking its best, to care for it on a daily basis, and to protect it. You'll also find tips for handling skin changes as you age.

✔ **Part II, "Hair":** Every woman's pet peeve is her hair. Whether it's finding the right hair color, the right styling products, or even the right style, hair care confuses all of us. In this part of the book, I cover everything you need to know in a language that you can understand.

✔ **Part III, "Makeup":** This part covers everything from basic makeup application to getting creative and experimenting. I include tips on finding the right tools, shaping your eyebrows, and choosing the colors and formulas that will work for you. There's also a full-color section that I've designed with the help of makeup artist and photographer François Nars to inspire you no matter what your look or age.

✔ **Part IV, "Home Spa":** This little part is big on indulgence. Here, I give you my secrets for turning your bathroom into a home spa where you can pamper your face, body, and hair. I also include step-by-step instructions for a professional-looking home manicure and pedicure.

✔ **Part V, "The Part of Tens":** This part has specific shopping tips, with my favorite brands named, as well as quick tips for varying your look with the products you already own.

This book also contains two useful appendixes. Appendix A is a glossary of more than 100 beauty terms (now you'll finally know what your colorist means when she talks about demipermanent color!). The book ends with a valuable list of beauty resources, found in Appendix B.

Icons Used in This Book

Throughout this book, you'll find icons beside certain paragraphs. These icons alert you to tips or other pieces of information that you don't want to miss.

If you see this icon, tread lightly and read carefully: The paragraph contains information that can save you from a beauty disaster or, worse, a potential health hazard.

Sometimes, you really need to see a doctor. This icon alerts you to situations that routine, at-home care doesn't cover. It also steers you toward information that comes straight from a dermatologist.

Beauty is expensive business, but you can cut back on your spending without compromising on quality. This icon points out those places where you can save a few extra dollars.

Like its name says, this icon alerts you to a beauty tip that will save you time, headaches, or both. As an added bonus, you'll get advice directly from pros who are currently working in the beauty industry.

This book is full of inside tips and beauty secrets from the experts and from me. But this icon draws your attention to tricks and techniques that I use myself and to routines that I follow personally.

Where to Go from Here

The beauty of this book is that you can jump in anywhere you choose — hair, skin, or makeup. I'll be there waiting with all my best beauty secrets.

Part I
Skin Care

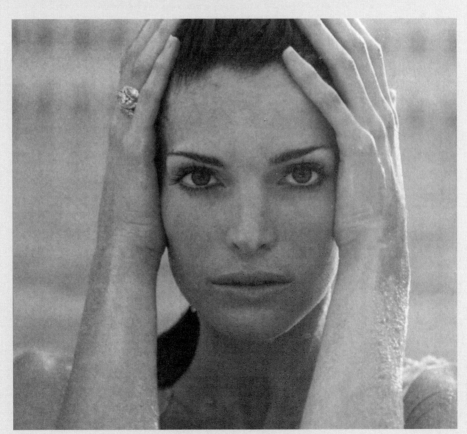

In this part . . .

Having beautiful skin, whatever your age may be, always boosts your confidence. When your skin is at its best, that healthy glow may be all you need to face the world. But many women feel that their skin looks less than perfect most of the time.

This part paves your way to better-looking skin. Here, you'll find information about determining your skin type; daily cleansing, exfoliating, and moisturizing; and doing those little extras to help your face look its very best. With the help of expert dermatologists, I also answer an array of questions about skin and skin care.

Chapter 1
Skin Basics

· ·

In This Chapter

▶ Understanding how skin works

▶ Knowing how skin ages

▶ Daily dos and don'ts for healthy skin

▶ Keeping your skin beautiful at any age

· ·

*I*n the never-ending quest for clearer, softer, smoother skin, it's easy to forget that skin's true function is to protect you from the outside world. The body's largest organ — about 20 square feet, in fact — your skin acts as your own personal suit of armor to shield you from the damaging effects of sun, pollution, smoke, weather, and water. It's also a mirror of what's going on *inside* you, showing the results of stress, diet, hormones, and health changes almost as quickly as they happen.

This chapter gives you the inside story on skin: how it functions, how it ages, and how a little common sense can keep your skin looking good throughout your lifetime.

How Skin Works

Your skin's outer layer — the one you see when you look in the mirror — is the *epidermis*. New skin cells are produced here, pushing up from the bottom (or *basal*) layer to the top in a continuous process of renewal. In younger women, this process may take as little as two weeks; for older women, the process can take twice as long. Most skin care products (other than prescription medications) work on this topmost layer only.

The *dermis* is the skin's thicker underlayer. Found in this level are the skin's *sebaceous* (or oil) glands, sweat glands, nerve endings, and blood vessels, plus stored water and fat. Also in the dermis are special cells that produce the skin's *melanin* — the substance that determines your natural skin tone and turns your skin darker when you tan. Even though you don't see the dermis, you do see the effect it has on your skin's appearance because the skin's natural *collagen* and *elastin* are located here. Responsible for skin's resilience and flexibility, both these fibers are vitally important for healthy-looking skin: When they degenerate from exposure to UV rays or the effects of normal aging, the result is wrinkles and loss of elasticity.

How Skin Ages

Aging of the skin is inevitable — but that doesn't mean that you're power-less over how aged your skin will look. Most of the signs we associate with growing older can be traced to two distinct factors:

✔ **Normal aging** occurs over the course of your lifetime, and how "old" you look in your later years is largely a matter of genetics. Over a period of decades, the skin gradually grows thinner, renews itself less often, produces less oil, and shows wrinkles. Blood vessels decrease in number and natural pigment fades, making skin appear lighter and providing less protection against the sun. Collagen and elastin break down, and the loss of elasticity, combined with the shifting and dissipation of the fat stores beneath the skin, results in contour changes in the cheeks, neck, jaw, and eye area.

✔ **Photoaging** is the one aspect of skin aging over which you *do* have total control. The sun is *the* most potent accelerator of aging, and years of repeated sun exposure can prompt the signs of normal aging to appear decades before they're due. The sun's UV rays speed the destruction of the skin's natural collagen and elastin, causing skin to develop very deep creases and a thick, leathery texture not common in normal aging. UV rays are also responsible for age spots and dilated blood vessels (not to mention 95 percent of all skin cancers). Wearing sunscreen every day helps to protect your skin from the sun's damaging effects.

Everyday Dos and Don'ts

Beyond the daily cleansing that's needed to keep skin healthy and clear (see Chapter 2 for more information about that), certain maintenance measures can have a real impact on your looks. They may require a bit of time and thought at first, but make them a part of your day-to-day routine and you'll see results — skin that looks fresh, smooth, and healthy — now and later in life.

Wear sunscreen

Wearing sunscreen every day is the best way to preserve your skin. As I explained earlier in this chapter, the sun is *the* primary cause of skin damage, accelerated aging, and skin cancer. Even if you're going to be outside for only a few minutes, protecting your skin with an SPF 15 (or higher) product is an absolute must. Every little bit adds up: Ten minutes of daily exposure over the course of a year equals a week of eight-hour days spent in the sun. "People don't realize that they have to wear sunscreen all the time, and not just when they're at the beach," says dermatologist Patricia Wexler, M.D. "You can get sun damage while driving your car if you're not wearing a sunblock with adequate protection."

You're also smart to avoid prolonged exposure during the hours of 10 a.m. and 3 p.m., when the sun's rays are strongest, and to wear a hat and sun-glasses to shield your face and sensitive eye area from the sun.

Drink plenty of water

Drinking six to eight glasses of water a day helps to keep the skin hydrated and moist, with a more supple appearance — especially helpful for dry skin. It also helps the body recover from the dehydrating effects of exercise, alcohol, or diet, and flushes out cellular wastes more efficiently. Taking in that much water can take some getting used to, so try building up one glass at a time (one glass on Monday, two on Tuesday, and so on) until you reach an amount that works for you. Remember: Other types of drinks don't count toward your total, especially soda, coffee, tea, or other beverages that contain dehydrating caffeine.

Throughout the day, I force myself to drink water rather than tea, coffee, soda, or juice. That way, I get the amount of water I need to maintain healthy skin and a healthy body. In the winter, no matter how much water I drink and no matter how much I moisturize my skin, it's still dry. Putting a humidifier in my bedroom keeps the air from robbing so much moisture from my skin.

Don't smoke

The message is right there in the Surgeon General's warning: Smoking causes cancer. If that's not enough to dissuade you, listen to this: Smoking also causes fine, feathery lines to form around your lip area, constricts blood vessels, inhibits oxygen delivery to the skin, prompts breakouts of adult acne, and discolors your pores and teeth. This habit takes a real toll on your looks — not to mention your health.

I know that some young girls are still drawn to smoking because they think it will help them stay thin, or look older or cooler, but there's absolutely nothing cool or glamorous about smoking or what it does to your looks.

Watch what you eat

Yes, eating healthy foods is common sense: A diet that's low in fat and that includes plenty of fruits, vegetables, and whole grains supplies the nutrients that keep the skin — and the entire body — in optimum condition. What's not as well-known is that maintaining a stable weight through proper diet and exercise is also important for preserving your skin's appearance. Repeated gains and losses mean that your skin must repeatedly grow and shrink. In later life especially, the results are stretch marks, wrinkling, and loose skin.

Some women may need to avoid certain foods and beverages. According to dermatologist Patricia Wexler, M.D., anything that makes the skin flush — shellfish, spicy foods, caffeine (including sodas and chocolate), and red wine — can exacerbate adult acne, also known as *rosacea* (see Chapter 3 for more on acne). Try eliminating these breakout triggers from your diet if rosacea's a problem for you.

Orange juice is something that I steer completely clear of. You may need to do so as well if you find that drinking it makes you break out like it does me. If I drink one glass of orange juice, I break out the next day — the high acid content causes it. Knowing this, I stay away from all high-acid drinks.

Exercise regularly

When it comes to exercise, most women concentrate on the total-body benefits that it gives — cardiovascular fitness, enhanced muscle tone, and weight maintenance — without realizing its importance in keeping the skin fit as well. Exercise increases blood flow to the skin (which is why your face flushes during a workout), nourishing cells with oxygen and nutrients, removing cellular wastes, and encouraging skin to work at maximum efficiency. Aerobic exercise of any type — walking, swimming, bicycling — gives the circulation a boost and is also one of the best ways to relieve stress (see "Limit stress" a little later in this chapter).

Avoid alcohol

Alcohol has two undesirable effects of the skin. First, it's highly dehydrating (which is why you crave water the morning after a big night out), robbing water from body tissues — including the skin, which makes wrinkles and undereye puffiness look more pronounced. Secondly, alcohol dilates the blood vessels; repeated expansion and contraction reduces their ability to shrink back to normal size, leaving your skin blotchy and red with small, visible veins. Over time, the veins can become increasingly swollen, notice-able — and permanent.

Here's one of my mother's favorite quotes about drinking, "You'd be better off washing your face in vodka than drinking it."

Limit stress

A certain amount of stress is inescapable: work, family, and money concerns are a never-ending part of life. The problem comes when stress is constant and at a high level. Not only can it contribute to skin-wreckers like insomnia (and other unhealthy habits like smoking, drinking, and unbalanced eating), but stress also prompts the body to increase its production of hormones — one of the primary causes of skin problems. You may never eliminate stress from your life completely, so you need to find a healthy way to *relieve* it. Exercise, meditation, massage, yoga, and relaxing baths (see Appendix A) are all wonderful ways to manage the stress of everyday life.

Get enough sleep

Easier said than done sometimes, but keeping a regular schedule with adequate sleep is crucial for helping the skin function efficiently and keeping those dark circles at bay (not to mention essential for your physical and mental well-being). Sleep-time is when the body finally has time to repair itself from the rigors of the day: When you're sleep-deprived, the body is unable to perform its nightly tune-up as quickly or completely.

I often suffer from insomnia when I'm working a lot, and it definitely affects my looks, not to mention my state of mind. Rather than take a sleeping pill, for me, the best way to deal with sleeping problems is to get a massage before I go to sleep. If you can't get a massage, a warm bath with plenty of Epsom salts and a little lavender oil is always soothing and prepares the body to rest.

Looking Great at Any Age

No matter what your age may be, keeping your skin in the best possible condition always gives you a healthy, more beautiful glow. At every stage of your life, you'll need to adapt your regimen, introducing new things, taking away things that don't work for you anymore, and basically just being aware of what's going on with your skin. The following sections define the stages and how to deal with them.

Teens

Hormones are in overdrive during the teen years, resulting in increased oil production — and the potential for breakouts. According to dermatologist Patricia Wexler, M.D., "At this age, it's important to have a good cleanser and to treat any acne problems." She recommends over-the-counter products containing salicylic acid or benzoyl peroxide for keeping breakouts in check (see Chapter 2 for more on these products). If you see no improvement, says Wexler, "You should really consider going to a physician because you don't want to leave scars in the skin." Dermatologists have an array of prescription medications that can clear up acne quickly and completely, so you have no reason to suffer through years of bad skin.

✔ Sun protection is vital for young skin: It's estimated that 80 percent of sun damage is done to the skin before age 20. If getting a tan is important to you or you spend a lot of time playing sports in the sun, opt for a sunblock with an SPF of at least 8 to 10 (SPF 20 is optimal). Keep in mind that a little sun on the face, as long as you have some protection, is perfectly fine; it's continual sunburns that do serious damage.

I always broke out from sunscreen. If the same thing happens to you, opt for a gel sunscreen (Shade makes a gel sunblock), which won't clog your pores. If that doesn't work, get used to wearing a baseball cap or some other sort of hat.

✔ Make sure to use a clean washcloth each time you wash your face. If you're having problems with your skin, bacteria from already-used washclothes may be the problem.

✔ Carry mild astringent pads with you so that you can freshen your face as needed throughout the day — a great way to cut down on shine and keep your pores clear when you aren't able to wash your face.

✔ Treat breakouts on your chest, back, and arms just as you would those on your face: Keep the area as clean as possible without overdrying, and apply an acne-control product to help keep blemishes at bay.

Twenties

In your twenties, it's time to get a little bit more sophisticated with your skin care regimen. The lucky ones had their bouts with acne in their teen years, but some unlucky women in their twenties suffer from adult acne due to hormones, pregnancy, or birth control pills. If your skin suddenly seems out of control, you may want to work with a dermatologist to get it back in the clear.

✔ Skin "grows up" during your twenties, so don't stick with your teen routine out of habit: The products that kept your skin under control at 16 may be too harsh now. Pay attention to skin's changes — and change your regimen accordingly.

✔ Slight irregularities in texture and tone can show up from past sun exposure. If your skin's not looking as fresh as you'd like, dermatologist Patricia Wexler, M.D., recommends "little refresher peels with either salicylic acid or alpha-hydroxy acids to give the skin a maintained glow." (See Chapter 3 for more on chemical peels.)

✔ You're mature enough now to handle a serious skin regimen, which must include gentle exfoliating treatments and soothing or moisturizing masks if you need them.

✔ You may or may not need a light moisturizer; use your best judgment.

✔ Eye creams and gels become important and useful at this stage in your life. As the eye-area skin becomes drier, you'll need to use an eye cream. For puffiness and dark circles, you need an eye gel.

Thirties

During your thirties, you certainly see fewer breakouts, but you begin to see the first signs of aging. Fine, dry lines usually begin to show around the eyes, where skin is at its thinnest. Overall, the skin is drier and slightly less elastic than it once was, which can result in light furrows on the forehead and between the eyes and "smile lines" around the mouth. This is normally the right time to start a skin regimen that includes light concentrations of glycolic acid or Retin-A, which help reduce the appearance of fine lines and give the skin a smoother, more supple look.

✔ Don't let time restrictions keep you from doing right by your skin. Though job and family demands may leave you little room for pampering, everyone has five minutes for her skin in the morning and five minutes in the evening — that's all you really need.

✔ You may notice that your pores look bigger than they used to: This stems from decreased elasticity in the skin. Although you can't shrink pores, you can minimize their appearance by keeping your skin very clean and dusting on a little loose powder to create an even-looking surface.

✔ An occasional exfoliating mask, followed by a moisturizing mask, is an instant freshen-up for your skin.

✔ Your day moisturizer may not be enough to keep your skin hydrated, especially in a dry climate or during the winter months when skin is driest. You may need to use a richer cream in the evenings if your skin still feels dry.

✔ Eye-area dryness makes eye cream a necessity, especially under your makeup: It helps to smooth and plump parched skin, making everything from concealer to shadow apply and adhere better. Eye gels help reduce puffiness and darkness under the eyes.

Forties

During your forties, you see noticeable changes in your skin's tone and texture: diminished elasticity, uneven pigmentation, and more pronounced creases — especially on the forehead and around the eyes. Hormone production decreases throughout this decade, prompting your skin to produce less and less oil; you may find yourself with dry skin for the first time in your life, and moisturizer becomes a must. Overall, skin doesn't bounce back as it once did, so conscientious daily care is more important than ever.

✔ Everything in your skin care regimen — cleanser, moisturizer, eye cream — should now be hydrating rather than drying.

✔ A few age spots and spider veins may appear on your face or hands, the result of years of exposure to the sun. Don't despair — they're easy to correct. (See Chapter 3 to find out how.)

✔ According to dermatologist Patricia Wexler, M.D., many women in their forties are ready for some sort of dermatological procedure to freshen up and immediately rejuvenate the skin. These procedures are usually non-invasive and require very little recovery time. Chapter 3 gives a brief overview of the latest rejuvenation procedures.

✔ Many women in their forties develop rosacea, a condition that can often look confusingly like acne (see Chapter 3 for more information). A dermatologist can treat this condition.

Fifties

In this decade, all you've done (or haven't done) to your skin makes itself known. You should by now have a skin care regimen that includes some type of daily exfoliating agent, such as glycolic acid, AHAs, or Retin-A, to keep the skin as smooth as possible. In your fifties, a suntan definitely only ages you and your skin and increases the size of any age spots you may already have. Minimizing the damaging effects of the sun by wearing sunscreen and/or a hat is a necessity.

✔ Because bodily processes slow down during these years, regular exercise is important: Revving up your circulation speeds oxygen and essential nutrients to the skin cells, helping them function at greater efficiency — and giving you a healthy-looking glow.

✔ The hormonal changes associated with menopause may cause unexpected breakouts, but flare-ups are usually short-lived. A mild-strength over-the-counter blemish cream keeps the occasional pimple in check.

- Many women in their fifties start thinking about face lifts. If you're not ready or willing to go that far, you may want to consider a laser peel, collagen injection, or Botox — all non-invasive procedures. See Chapter 3 for more information about the various procedures that are available.

- The incidence of skin cancer is greater during this decade; diligent self-examination, plus twice-yearly skin exams by your dermatologist, are a must for early detection. (See Chapter 3 for more information about skin cancer.)

Sixties and up

In your sixties, your eyelids droop, your undereye bags become more pronounced, and your facial lines deepen and become more plentiful. Your skin is probably the palest it's ever been, making pigmentation irregularities more noticeable. The best thing you can do for your skin now is to focus on getting your skin tone as even as possible. Obviously, you're going to have wrinkles, and obviously, you're going to look more mature. Enjoy your skin at this age, stay out of the sun, and keep your skin well moisturized so that it retains a soft, smooth texture. Older skin can still be beautiful — so give yourself the attention you deserve.

- Your thinner, lighter skin burns very easily when exposed to the sun. In addition to a high-SPF sunscreen, wear a hat to further shield your face and scalp, and cover exposed areas (arms, shoulders, and legs) with clothing whenever you're outdoors.

- If you're interested in smoothing your skin texture or decreasing the appearance of age spots, see a dermatologist.

- Some sort of non-invasive procedure to tighten the skin's appearance can give you an extra boost of confidence for special occasions. (See Chapter 2 for more information.)

- Eye creams help keep dry eye-area skin hydrated. If eye puffiness is a problem, the same eye gel you used when you were younger is still effective for reducing puffiness now.

Chapter 2

Caring for Your Skin

•••

•••

Caring for your skin is the most important step in your beauty regimen. Over the years, I've gone through many battles with my own skin, as I'm sure you have, unless you're one of the lucky few who just have perfect skin no matter what you do. The most common skin dilemmas stem from hormonal changes, sun damage, and using the wrong makeup or skin care products.

The idea behind any skin care routine is to analyze your skin and give it what it needs. Says dermatologist Patricia Wexler, M.D., "You need four basic things to take care of your skin. You need a gentle cleanser, you have to exfoliate in some form on a regular basis, you need a moisturizer, and you need a sunscreen." In this chapter, I help you decide what type of cleanser, exfoliant, moisturizer, and sunscreen are right for your skin type. The following section can help you determine your skin type.

Finding Your Skin Type

Maybe you have a pretty good idea of what skin type you have — but did you know that using the wrong skin care products can disguise your skin's true tendencies? Harsh treatment of normal skin makes it seem dry, while inadequate cleansing of combination skin can make it seem oilier than it really is. Remember, too, that your skin is always changing — whether slightly or substantially — in response to shifts in hormones, weather, diet, and other factors.

To get a true picture of your skin, do this simple test: In the morning when your skin's makeup-free, wash your face with a mild cleanser, pat it dry, and then do nothing else to your skin for an hour. After an hour, check your face in the mirror and then press the corners of a clean facial tissue onto your forehead, nose, chin, and cheeks.

- ✔ You have **normal skin** if your skin shows no overly shiny spots, feels comfortable, and leaves no residue on the tissue. Thank your lucky genes if you have this easy-to-care-for skin type.

- ✔ You have **combination skin** if your *T-zone* (forehead, nose, and chin) is shiny and shows oil on the tissue, and your cheeks are normal. Combination skin is very common.

- ✔ You have **oily or acne-prone skin** if your entire face is shiny when you look in the mirror, and all four facial areas leave oil on the tissue. Oily skin usually can be traced to hormones.

- ✔ You have **dry skin** if your skin looks tight or flaky, feels uncomfortable, and deposits no oil on the tissue (and perhaps leaves a few skin flakes instead). Dry skin results when the skin doesn't produce enough oils to retain its own natural moisture.

- ✔ There's no agreed-upon definition of **sensitive skin**, and the truth is that most women — dry, normal, combination, and oily alike — have adverse reactions to products from time to time. Signs of sensitivity can range from dry, flaky patches to red bumps to raised, itchy areas; some skins react to one certain ingredient, and others are irritated even by plain tap water.

Cleansing

Cleansing, perhaps the most important step in the skin care routine, is also the step that's most often done incorrectly. The idea is to remove all traces of makeup, excess oil, dirt, and dead cells without leaving a residue or stripping the skin. Most dermatologists recommend a cleanser that is water-soluble, which rinses off completely and doesn't irritate the eyes. They also suggest using tepid water; hot water can burn the skin, and cold water shocks it.

After an exhausting day (or a fabulous night out), you may feel tempted to break the rules and skip washing your face. A word of advice: Don't. It isn't worth it. At the very least, cleanse your skin and skip the other steps.

Facial cleansers

Today's cleansers don't just remove surface dirt and oil. Now they protect the face and give it radiance by adding vitamins, antioxidants, emollients, and exfoliants. You can find a cleanser for every skin type listed here:

- **Foaming cleansers** are gentle enough for normal skin but strong enough to handle an oilier T-zone.

- **Gel cleansers** are virtually oil-free and are less alkaline than soap. They may contain AHAs or BHA, and they also rinse off easily. Gels are recommended for oily and combination skin.

- **Lotion cleansers** are good for dry or sensitive skin because they contain milder surfactants and moisturizers and leave a light film on the skin that soothes dry or sensitive skin.

- **Water-soluble cleansers**, such as Cetaphil, are good all-purpose cleansers for all skin types. They are non-irritating, which makes them good for general cleansing.

- **Cleansing milks** come in three forms, with ingredients based on skin type: normal, combination, or oily.

- **Oil-free cleansing lotions** often contain glycolic acid and are good for combination skin.

Find your skin type in Table 2-1 to determine what type of cleanser is best for you.

Table 2-1   Cleansers Recommended for Various Skin Types

Skin Type	Cleansing Ritual
Normal	A gentle, water-soluble cleanser or a cleansing milk
Oily or acne-prone	A gel or lotion cleanser containing salicylic acid to clear out the bacteria build-up that leads to breakouts
Combination	A foaming cleanser or cleansing lotion with salicylic acid; focus on the T-zone while cleansing
Dry	A gentle cleansing milk or water-soluble cleanser; look for products that leave the skin clean, with a light, emollient film on the surface to soothe dry skin
Sensitive	A gentle, water-soluble cleanser or a cleansing milk made for sensitive skin

Soaps

Soap is the most basic form of cleanser. The problem with traditional soaps is that they can be too alkaline for most skins. The skin is slightly acidic, with a pH of about 5 to 6, but the pH of most bar soaps is about 10. The change in the skin's pH can leave a tight, uncomfortable feeling. Unless your dermatologist has recommended a particular medicated soap for a specific skin condition, you're better off to stick with the cleansers mentioned earlier in this chapter.

Makeup removers

Most facial cleansers will remove a normal amount of makeup, although not all are good for removing eye makeup; anything harsh or drying will irritate and slowly deteriorate the eye area skin. If your cleanser doesn't say that it removes eye makeup, don't use it for that purpose. For removing heavy makeup, use a makeup remover or a mild, creamy cleanser and then cleanse as you normally do.

Skin-cleansing tipsheet

✔ Cleanse and then moisturize your face twice daily.

✔ When you've used heavy makeup, make sure to cleanse your face with a makeup remover and then your cleanser, twice if necessary.

✔ Always use a soft washcloth or cotton pads dampened with tepid water to get the first layer of cleanser off your face, and then splash your face several times with tepid water to make sure that all the product has been thoroughly rinsed off your skin.

Exfoliating

Exfoliants slough off excess cells from the skin surface and can make your skin look smoother by exposing the newer skin cells hiding underneath the old ones. Regular exfoliation also helps your skin absorb moisturizers better and allows makeup to cover more smoothly.

"Exfoliating gives the skin a healthy glow and gets rid of those spots that tend to make us look fallow and our skin look blotchy or irregular," says dermatologist Patricia Wexler, M.D. "It works for acne and fine lines and is also great for keeping the skin looking fresh."

The range of products used for exfoliating is incredibly vast. An exfoliant can be as simple as a washcloth or as high-tech as the latest serums that contain alpha-hydroxy acids (AHAs). The most important thing to remember when choosing your formula is what you want. Either you use an exfoliating mask weekly just to keep your skin looking as fresh as possible, or you use an exfoliating cleanser or serum to help clear up acne, clean up your skin's texture and coloration, and reduce the look of fine lines.

- **Silk mitts or synthetic loofahs** are manual exfoliants that you use to gently scrub off dead skin cells. "Using a silk mitt while you're cleansing is preferable to using a natural loofah on the face," Wexler says. "Natural loofahs are usually abrasive and too strong. But you can get synthetic loofahs that are smooth and just use movement to exfoliate dead cells."

- **Exfoliating masks** are massaged in, left on for a short time, and then rinsed off. This type of mask is best for normal or sensitive skin.

- **Facial scrubs** contain tiny particles that loosen dead skin cells. They come in gel and cleanser forms and are massaged onto the skin and then rinsed off. When you rinse off the scrub, the old skin cells are washed away.

- **Buffing creams** are left on for five to ten minutes and then sloughed off in a circular motion. They are usually more effective at exfoliating than facial scrubs.

Because overly harsh exfoliating scrubs and buffing creams can cause broken capillaries and irritation in sensitive skin, it's best to choose a product with a light texture and fine, even particles. Natural abrasives are no better than synthetic ones — natural ingredients such as peach pits can be irregularly shaped and irritating. These products must be used gently and should be kept away from the eye area.

- **AHAs,** or fruit acids, work as exfoliators. They are commonly found in a new breed of exfoliators that include gels, lotions, and even facial masks.

- **Tretinoin**, a chemical exfoliator, is a prescription formula of vitamin A-derived solutions (with the brand names Retin-A and Renova) that help your skin shed cells. On the surface, tretinoin exfoliates by dissolving the top layer of the skin. The downside is that tretinoin solutions can be irritating to sensitive and dry skin. This product should be used under the supervision of a dermatologist.

Remember that both AHAs and tretinoin can be very drying. If you're using products that contain these ingredients, make sure to use a good moisturizer.

Be gentle

"Scrubbing is for floors, not skin," says dermatologist Patricia Wexler, M.D. Any shopper who enters a drugstore and finds pads, nylon net puffs, loofahs, fiber or nylon mitts, and brushes for exfoliating the skin should keep that statement in mind. Most manual exfoliators are too abrasive and irritating and are hard to keep clean. If you're prone to red pimples (called *inflammatory acne*), avoid rubbing to exfoliate, and consult a dermatologist if acne persists.

Table 2-2 tells you which exfoliants are best for each skin type.

Table 2-2   Exfoliants Recommended for Various Skin Types

Skin Type	Exfoliating Ritual
Normal	Use a washcloth, an exfoliating rub-off mask, or an AHA product.
Oily or acne-prone	Exfoliate with an AHA product to avoid scrubbing, which can irritate skin and cause acne flare-ups.
Combination	Use any of the exfoliants recommended for normal or oily/acne-prone skin.
Dry	Use a gentle exfoliant such as a washcloth or silk mitt or a massage-in and wash-off exfoliating mask such as an oatmeal mask.
Sensitive	Because exfoliating can cause broken capillaries and irritation in sensitive skin, stay away from buffing creams and facial scrubs. Use the gentlest exfoliant possible — a washcloth with your cleanser, a silk mitt, or an exfoliating mask.

Moisturizing

Moisturizers don't actually soak into your skin and replace moisture; they work by keeping your skin's natural moisture from evaporating by forming a barrier between the skin and the air. When you moisturize, you temporarily trap water in the skin, which plumps the skin and gives it a smoother appearance. Moisturizers provide relief from itchy, irritated skin as well. Many moisturizers also contain ingredients that help temporarily repair damaged skin. But be aware that if you have oily or acne-prone skin, moisturizer can clog pores.

No rule says that you have to use moisturizer all over your face; you may just need a light eye cream or a bit of moisturizer on your drier cheek area. You may need to change your moisturizer seasonally as well. Some women break out more often in hot, humid weather and must use oil-free products during the hot, sticky months. Others decide that they need moisturizer only in the winter.

Here's an easy way to tell whether you need moisturizer: Wash your face with a gentle cleanser, and then wait half an hour to see whether your skin produces enough oil to make it feel comfortable. If it still feels tight in some areas, you need to moisturize those areas.

✔ **Oil-free (lightweight lotions and gels):** If you're looking for an oil-free moisturizer, look for these ingredients: mucopolysaccharides and hyaluronic acid. Although they sound complex, these ingredients work simply because they are comprised of large molecules that can't be absorbed by the skin. As a result, they form a water-binding film on the skin's surface.

   Glycerin: A more familiar ingredient, glycerin is a humectant that attracts water and has long been used to hydrate chapped skin. It's also a common ingredient in oil-free moisturizers.

✔ **Moisturizers that contain oils:** Moisturizers use a vast array of oils, including vegetable oils, animal oils, and mineral oils. Even though plant oils such as macadamia oil and jojoba oil may sound more exotic than petroleum or mineral oil, all these oils are equally effective because they can be absorbed into the skin, allowing them to moisturize the epidermis.

In Table 2-3, you can find out which type of moisturizer will work best for your skin type.

Table 2-3 Moisturizers Recommended for Various Skin Types

Skin Type	Moisturizing Ritual
Normal	If you need a moisturizer, use a light, water-based formula.
Oily or acne-prone	Use an oil-free product, preferably in a gel form, only if needed on dry areas.
Combination	Because your skin tends to be oilier in parts, use a very lightweight, water-based moisturizer where needed.

(continued)

Table 2-3 *(continued)*

Skin Type	Moisturizing Ritual
Dry	Use a moisturizer with heavier emollients. You may even want to have two moisturizers: a very light one for the day, and a heavier one for deep moisturizing and relief at night.
Sensitive	Find a product with as few ingredients as possible to cut down your chances of irritation. Try spot-testing a light, fragrance-free, hypoallergenic moisturizer.

Hytone, an extremely light prescription hydrocortisone lotion, is something I always keep in my medicine cabinet. It's wonderful to have when your skin is irritated for any reason and you need something to soothe it, moisturize it, and take down the redness.

Eye creams

The theory behind eye cream is that because the skin around your eyes is more delicate than the rest of the skin on your face, you need a different moisturizing product for that area. In truth, most facial products can be used around the eyes. However, if your eye area is drier than the rest of your skin, you will benefit from a more emollient cream.

Other than eye creams, you also can find eye gels, which are lighter in weight. Being less emollient, their purpose is not solely to moisturize but to reduce puffiness as well.

I recommend having an eye cream and an eye gel, because eye cream is essential on a daily basis to keep the skin around your eyes looking smooth, and eye gel is used on those days when you have undereye puffiness.

Dating all the way back to the 1950s, many makeup artists have used Preparation H cream or ointment underneath movie stars' eyes to control puffiness, add moisture, and tighten the skin. This is, of course, not recommended on a daily basis, but used sparingly, it does work wonders for a special night out.

Skin care boosters defined

As I've mentioned in various descriptions in this chapter, many skin care products contain "extras" that help improve skin's appearance. In case you're wondering what these extras are, here are some definitions:

- **AHAs and BHA:** Glycolic (sugar cane), citric (fruits), malic (apples), and lactic (mild) acids. These ingredients, found in everything from facial cleansers to masks to body lotions, work by promoting the exfoliation of the skin's outer layer of cells, which stimulates newer, fresher cells to come to the surface faster. Most over-the-counter products contain about 2 percent. Don't overuse AHAs and BHA: Try them in a cream or serum form, which stays on the skin longer. AHA and BHA products can also be found in prescription strength. They are used in peels done by dermatologists as well.

- **Antioxidants (free-radical fighters):** These chemicals absorb or quench harmful molecules called *free radicals*. One theory is that the cumulative damage from free radicals leads to the physical deterioration known as aging. Antioxidants include the mineral selenium and vitamins A, C, and E. Although cosmetic companies have begun adding antioxidants to makeup, cleansers, moisturizers, sunscreens, and more, research is still underway to determine whether applying them topically really helps your skin.

- **Botanicals:** A fancy word for products extracted from plants.

- **Collagen and elastin:** These two substances are found in living skin, but their processed versions (usually from cows) are molecules that are much too large to penetrate the skin from the outside.

- **Humectants:** These moisturizing ingredients may draw water to the skin from the environment or from the dermis. Humectants may be used in oil-free preparations, which are recommended for acne-prone skin.

- **SPF:** Sunscreens are rated with an SPF (sun protection factor) that starts at 2 and goes up. Most dermatologists recommend an SPF of 15 or higher. Products with an SPF are the only ones that can claim to be anti-aging, because much of the aging that occurs in skin is due to sun exposure — not to getting older.

Sunscreen

Sunscreen formulas for the face have come a long way in the last few years. Advanced product technology has enabled companies to develop lightweight, comfortable formulas that are non-greasy, long-lasting, and less irritating.

Dermatologist Fred Brandt, M.D., believes that everyone can save a lot of money on skin care down the road by using sunscreen today. "My money-saving suggestion for people at a young age is to start to be careful of the sun and use sunscreens, because the sun is a primary cause of photoaging and damage to the skin," he says. "And it's also a health risk because of skin cancer. People don't realize that they have to wear sunscreen all the time, not just when they're at the beach. You get sun damage through the car window, you can get spotting, you can get the melasma or the pregnancy mask just by driving your car and not wearing a sunblock with adequate protection."

Many indoor tanning parlors advertise themselves to be safe alternatives to natural sunlight. The truth is that most indoor tanning devices work by generating UVA light, so you're actually being exposed to a concentrated dose of dangerous, skin-aging UVA rays. If you want a little color on your face, try a bronzer instead. (See Chapter 11.)

Very high SPF numbers can also be misleading. Tests have shown that an SPF 15 absorbs 93 percent of the sun's burning rays, while an SPF 30 product absorbs 97 percent. Any percentage gain after that point is considered negligible. In fact, the FDA has suggested that SPFs over 30 offer little additional benefit and may expose the consumer to unnecessarily high levels of chemicals.

I keep a cosmetic bag specifically with sunscreens in it, some for my body and some for my face. During the summer, when I'm going to the beach or the pool, I toss my bag of sunscreens into my beach bag so that I have a range of sunscreen products for my body and my face. Remember, whether you're fair or dark, the skin on your face and your chest is much more fragile and sensitive than the skin on the rest of your body, so use a sunscreen specifically formulated for the face on these areas and use an SPF of 15 or higher. Wearing a sunscreen of an SPF of 15 or higher is an absolute must. Don't worry; you'll still get sun.

Sunscreen tipsheet

- ✔ Because facial skin is more sensitive than the skin on the body, you must have a separate sunscreen that's made for use on the face.

- ✔ If facial sunscreens make your skin break out, don't just not use them. Speak with a dermatologist, who can help you find a sunscreen that's compatible with your skin type.

- ✔ Many foundations, tinted moisturizers, and lipsticks now come with SPF 15 protection, making them ideal daily-wear options for protecting your skin against incidental sun exposure.

- ✔ Your skin type should guide you in your choice of formula; look for oil-free gels or sprays if you have breakout-prone skin, creamier formulas if your skin tends to be dry. If you have sensitive skin, try a sunscreen that's specially formulated for babies.

- ✔ Choose a high SPF and reapply sunscreen often, especially after swimming, sweating, or toweling off. (Waterproof formulas last longest.)

- ✔ Apply sunscreen 30 minutes before sun exposure to give your skin time to fully absorb it. Put it on before you get dressed so that you don't miss any areas.

- ✔ You won't get full protection if you spread sunscreen too thin. To make sure that you're getting the protection you need, choose a lightweight formula that still feels comfortable and looks natural on the skin even if you apply a fairly generous amount.

- ✔ The skin around your eyes is the thinnest and most vulnerable on the face, so protection is vital. Any sunscreen you use in the immediate eye area should be made for that specific purpose. Look for formulas that do not contain fragrance or other common irritants, that are matte-textured or waterproof so as not to run into eyes, and that are ophthalmologist-tested.

- ✔ Lips are a common site for skin cancer, and sunlight also stimulates the reemergence of cold sores. Get into the habit of wearing an SPF 15 lipstick or lip balm every day. An SPF 15 lip balm also works in a pinch for spot-protection of your nose, ear tops, or other areas.

- ✔ Wear sunglasses that block UVA and UVB rays, and remember that wearing eye-area sunblock is still important: Sunglasses protect your eyes but have not been shown to protect skin.

MEDICAL MATTERS

Sunscreen prescribed

You *must* use sunscreen without fail if

- ✔ **You're using Retin-A or Renova.** These two topical medications can thin the skin, making it more susceptible to burning.

- ✔ **You've had a facial chemical peel.** Just-peeled skin is less able to defend itself from ultraviolet rays; exposure can also lead to uneven pigmentation — which may be one reason you had the peel in the first place!

- ✔ **You've had plastic surgery.** Exposing scars and fragile, post-surgical skin to sunlight can lead to thickening and permanent discoloration.

- ✔ **You're taking certain medications that sensitize your skin to the sun.** ChJck with your doctor or pharmacist to find out whether you need to be extra-cautious of the sun because of a medication you're taking.

Skin Care Extras

When it comes to your skin looking its best, it's the little things that seem to matter most. This section gives you a few tips that can enhance the appearance of your skin and boost your confidence.

Masks

Dermatologists differ in their opinions of the effectiveness of facial masks, but I love them for keeping my skin fresh and drawing out impurities when necessary. Masks help clean pores and slough off dead cells. But don't abuse or overuse masks — a mask every couple of weeks is plenty. Used as a once-in-a-while treat, they can make your skin look and feel healthier.

Following are some common types of masks:

- ✓ **Clay:** This type of mask dries on the skin. Deep-cleansing clay or mud masks soak up oil, draw out impurities, and tighten pores. Ingredients may include corn or wheat starch, charcoal, or titanium dioxide to increase the mask's drying properties. This type of mask can be applied over the entire face or just over the T-zone, where oil may be more prominent.

- ✓ **Moisturizing:** Moisturizing masks are usually creamy and work well on dry or normal skin by bringing in a mixture of moisture and nutrients. The cream or gel base provides a barrier to help skin retain its own natural moisture.

- ✓ **Soothing:** A gel- or cream-based mask with anti-inflammatory ingredients such as algae, azulene, or chamomile can relieve irritated skin. A gel is best for oily or sensitive skin, while a cream-based mask works well for dry skin.

Topical blemish medicines

Over-the-counter products, tinted or not, can camouflage blemishes and heal them at the same time. They are typified by their active ingredient:

- ✓ **Benzoyl peroxide:** This disinfectant and drying agent is often used to fight acne.

- ✓ **Salicylic acid:** This beta-hydroxy acid and mild exfoliant can be helpful in drying up blemishes.

If you're out of blemish medicine, you can use a dot of a clay or other drying mask instead.

Toners and astringents

You may love the pleasantly fresh, tingly feeling that toners and astringents leave on your skin. But if a product is overly drying, your skin will produce more oil later on. Toners and astringents remove surface skin cells, soap residue, and oils from the skin. Although not necessary on a daily basis, they're nice to have in the cabinet on hot, muggy days for oilier skin types, to keep in your gym bag, or just to be used when you need to take an extra measure to be sure that your skin is thoroughly cleansed.

- **Toners:** Toners return the skin to its natural pH after you use a more emollient cleanser. Be careful with toners that contain witch hazel or alcohol; these can be very drying, although women with oily skin types may find their drying properties balancing.

- **Astringents and clarifying lotions:** These products usually contain alcohol, which can be very drying to all but the oiliest skins. Use with caution, and only when it's really called for — when your skin is very oily during the summer months, or after a rigorous workout.

Facial facts

When done well, facials can feel wonderful. But dermatologists say that the results are more relaxing than actually beneficial to the skin. The deep-cleansing effects of a facial last only a few days. Facialists, however, contend that a regular facial gets rid of dead cells that accumulate in the natural cycle of skin growth, although if you're exfoliating on a regular basis at home, you're doing the same thing that they're doing without the extra cost. If you enjoy facials and don't experience side effects such as breakouts, they're probably harmless, so relax and enjoy.

Most facials involve

- Cleaning off makeup
- Analyzing the skin
- Steaming to open pores
- Deep-cleaning through extraction
- Massaging
- Applying a light exfoliant peel
- Applying at least one mask that's appropriate for your skin type
- Hydrating with an appropriate moisturizer

If the steam is too hot or the facialist or any of the products being used on your skin is making you uncomfortable or hurting you, say so immediately. By speaking up, you help your facialist avoid irritating your skin by using the wrong techniques or products. A facialist shouldn't hard-sell you on products, but many salons or facialists do have products of a very high quality that aren't always available through other outlets.

Exploring Skin Care Sources

There's certainly no shortage of sales outlets for skin care products. You can purchase them at an array of places, including drugstores, beauty supply stores, health food stores, department stores, and day spas.

Purchasing skin care products from a drugstore, beauty supply store, or health food store is generally more of a do-it-yourself approach than a visit to a department store or day spa is. That's not all bad, especially if you're an informed shopper. Despite the expertise that most salespeople in department stores and day spas are supposed to have, you still must buy products based on your knowledge of your own skin. Remember, most of these salespeople get a commission on what they sell, so if you're only trying to buy a cleanser and they're trying to sell you the entire skin care line, trust yourself and buy just the cleanser. If you love it and want to try more products, you can always call the store and have individual products sent to you, or you can take some samples home and try the products before you make a big investment in a whole skin care line.

Because you must rely on your own knowledge when buying skin care products from outlets such as drugstores, beauty supply stores, and specialty beauty care boutiques, remember to read the ingredient lists, and keep in mind any particular ingredients that don't agree with your skin. Look for the simplest products with the clearest labels as to which skin type they're for. If possible, ask a salesperson if you can try a little bit of the product on your hand or smell it. Doing so may give you an indication of whether it's right for you.

The way your skin looks has little to do with how much money you spend on skin care products; the most important thing is to find products that work with your skin type, leaving it looking fresh and smooth and never irritated. Finding the right products involves a lot of trial-and-error, so be patient.

Chapter 3
Beyond the Basics

· ·

In This Chapter

▶ Common skin problems and how to solve them

▶ Products and procedures that refresh skin's look

▶ Skin rejuvenation for the face

· ·

Skin problems come in a variety of forms — some perfectly harmless, some harmless-looking but quite serious. Distinguishing the differences by yourself is often difficult. This chapter gives you the facts on common skin problems, including what causes them and what fixes them. You'll also find out that sometimes you may need to see a dermatologist or plastic surgeon.

Building a relationship with a dermatologist is a good idea for anyone, especially a woman who cares about her skin. If you're in a small town, you may have to go to the city nearest you, but it's worth it — I drive an hour to my doctor myself. You can go a couple times a year to have your skin and moles checked, or you can go every few months and have a little tune-up to maintain your skin. A dermatologist can do so many non-invasive, non-surgical, and very safe things right in the office. If you tell the dermatologist what you're unhappy with, he or she can tell you what your options are, whether you're dealing with little broken veins on your legs, discoloration on your face, or scars from surgery or accidents. Or maybe your skin is always broken out or just isn't looking as fresh as it used to. Whatever your problem, a good dermatologist or plastic surgeon who specializes in skin as well as cosmetic surgery usually has a solution.

Solving Common Skin Problems

If you've ever awakened with a surprise pimple, you know that changes can occur in a matter of hours. But once you understand what's behind a skin problem, solving it is all the easier. This section provides a helpful listing of common skin complaints and the best ways to correct them.

Acne

Acne is a chronic inflammation of the skin's sebaceous (or oil) glands. It's believed to stem from a few causes: overactive oil glands stimulated by hormonal activity, oversensitivity to even normal levels of hormones, bacteria, and also genetics. *Cystic acne* occurs when a blocked pore ruptures deeply under the skin, causing an infection.

So how do you determine whether you have true acne? "My criteria are, 'Is it chronic, has it never been clear, and are you getting scars?'" says dermatologist Joel Kassamir, M.D. "If the answer to those three questions is yes, you most likely do have acne and need a dermatologist's help — especially if you're getting scars."

Although acne is most common in adolescence, it can also occur later in life — usually related to hormonal changes, stress, and even medications — so don't ignore bad skin simply because you think that you're too old for acne. Early, continued treatment by a dermatologist is the best approach to solving chronic acne problems.

Your dermatologist has many prescription treatments to offer, from oral antibiotics (tetracycline, doxycycline, or minocycline) to topical antibiotics (clindamycin or erythromycin) to injections of cortisone, which can make a pimple disappear in a day or two. You may need to use other medications, such as birth control pills or Accutane, if nothing else works. Women of childbearing age must discuss the pros and cons of oral acne medication with their physicians, as some can cause birth defects.

Accutane

When all else fails to clear up chronic acne, the prescription drug Accutane (isotretinoin) usually is called for. Says dermatologist Joel Kassamir, M.D., "Accutane seems to have an antibacterial effect, and it binds to the oil glands and sort of turns them off. I always tell patients that they have subway tunnels underneath their skin that harbor bacteria, and when you take Accutane it gives you a chance to heal."

In the past, Accutane had a somewhat scary reputation — related to the fact that patients must be monitored by blood tests throughout treatment, and that women must not become pregnant while using the drug — but many doctors are convinced that the benefits are worth it. "I would absolutely recommend Accutane rather than see a person develop scars that may need significant surgery," says dermatologist Patricia Wexler, M.D. "I think that there is a definite need to go through traditional forms of therapy first — antibiotics, topical medications, a change in hygiene — but for a teenager who's got severe inflammation of the skin and scarring, the damage that's done to self-esteem during those formative years is much worse than the damage done by a low dose of Accutane."

Together with your physician, you can decide whether Accutane is a good option for you.

Blemishes

Everyday blemishes develop when excess oil and dead skin cells clog pores. When this debris isn't able to exit smoothly, it forms a plug that can continue to grow, bacteria moves in and infects the pore, and voilà, you have a pimple. Hormones are a major contributor to blemishes because they stimulate excess oil production. Improper cleansing that leaves debris on the skin also can contribute to blocked pores.

Pore-related problems come in a few different forms:

- ✔ **Blackheads** are plugs that are open to the air at the skin's surface; exposure to the air is responsible for the dark color.

- ✔ **Whiteheads** are plugs of sebum that remain under the skin. When they continue to fill with sebum and cellular debris, they can rupture the pore and form a pimple.

- ✔ **Cysts** are small, enclosed deposits of cellular debris and sebum within the skin that show as bumps on skin's surface. They include *milia* (tiny cysts in the oil gland) and *follicular cysts* (at the hair root). Don't pick: Some may lose inflammation and go away on their own. If, after ten days, the inflammation hasn't gone down and the cyst is still full, see a dermatologist.

Over-the-counter blemish products, which are easily accessible at any drugstore, should do the trick. Dermatologist Joel Kassamir, M.D., recommends using a facial wash in combination with a spot-treatment gel, both formulated with benzoyl peroxide. "You get a global treatment, then a more focused treatment," he says. "Wash your face with a product at a 2 percent concentration of benzoyl peroxide — if it's not too drying, you can go to 5 percent — and then put the gel directly on the blemishes." If this treatment doesn't clear things up in a week or so, see a dermatologist.

To pick or not to pick

Dermatologists cringe at the thought, but they know that women have a hard time letting a pimple just sit there. "If the plug comes out easily after you've taken a shower when the pores are warm and open — well, all right," says dermatologist Joel Kassamir, M.D.

If I look in the mirror and see something that I really want to pick, I wait a week, because it always looks better when you don't pick it. Most times, it's a matter of using a blemish medicine to cover it up during the day.

Cold sores

These red, blistery sores (also known as fever blisters) usually occur around the mouth and are often accompanied by tingling or discomfort. Caused by the virus herpes simplex I, cold sores are highly contagious when they're open, so you *must* keep your hands away from them. Left untouched, sores should disappear in about a week.

Over-the-counter medications can help speed the healing of cold sores. Prescription drugs help treat new breakouts and can also be taken over a period of months to help prevent recurrences (see Chapter 4 for more information). But the best strategy is to avoid cold-sore triggers — and the prime culprit is sun exposure. Wear an SPF 15 lip balm daily and reapply often to keep sores at bay.

Collagen changes

Collagen is not only one of the building blocks of the skin; it's also one of its primary repair tools. Any time the skin is cut, burned, or otherwise injured, collagen covers the area to seal and strengthen it — but the repair work is often visible and less smooth than what surrounds it. Though collagen changes gradually fade and soften, certain treatments diminish their appearance more quickly.

Scars

Dozens of different skin injuries can cause scars, but scars typically appear in two basic types. In both cases, collagen forms at the injured area in a less-organized manner, leaving the skin with an obvious difference in texture.

- **Raised scars** usually result from deep wounds, such as surgical incisions. If they persist or are common in your family, seek immediate treatment.
- **Recessed scars** often appear after a bout with cystic acne or chicken pox.

Raised scars can be corrected with laser resurfacing or dermabrasion; recessed scars can be filled in with collagen or fat injections; very uneven skin textures (as with acne scarring) can benefit from a combination of both types of treatment. (See "Procedures" later in this chapter for more information about all these techniques.)

Keloids

Resulting from a pronounced overgrowth of tissue, keloids are much harder, thicker, and irregularly colored than the basic raised scar. Although dark-skinned women are particularly prone to keloids, many light-skinned women also develop these thickened scars; severe acne and surgery are typical causes. If you know that you're predisposed to keloid scarring, avoid picking at your skin, especially on the face. If you're contemplating a surgical procedure, be sure to discuss with your doctor specific incision placement prior to surgery and talk about what type of after-care will be used to keep scarring to a minimum.

Treatment of keloids includes injections of steroid medications, laser resurfacing, and silicone sheeting. For these treatments, see a dermatologist who specializes in these areas.

Pigmentation problems

Melanin, the substance that determines your skin color Nnd how you tan, is also linked to most skin discoloration problems. *Hypopigmentation,* which is the loss of melanin, is often due to genetics, skin resurfacing techniques, and just plain aging; *hyperpigmentation,* which is an overabundance of melanin, is usually traced to sun exposure, medications (including birth control pills), pregnancy, hormones, and age. Both conditions can take on many forms, so a dermatologist's evaluation is always advised.

- ✔ **Age spots:** Also known as lentigos or liver spots, these concentrated areas of pigment appear on areas of skin that have endured years of damaging sun exposure — usually the face, hands, and upper back. Heredity is also a contributing factor in some cases. Treatment options include over-the-counter or prescription skin-bleaching products, tretinoin, chemical peels, and laser correction. A dermatologist can also freeze off age spots.

- ✔ **Freckles:** Not a skin problem per se, unless you dislike them. Freckles are small specks of excess pigment that can appear all over the body but are much more evident on the face. Most freckles are genetically determined (think of the classic freckle-faced redhead), but sun exposure can make them intensify and multiply. If you're prone to freckles, wear sunscreen and avoid the sun. Skin-bleaching or tretinoin products may help fade very dark freckles. Skin-resurfacing procedures, although not recommended for this purpose alone, often result in lightened skin coloration, although you won't necessarily get more even color.

- ✔ **Melasma:** This condition is also known as the "mask of pregnancy" because darkened skin usually appears across the cheeks, forehead, and nose. The body's hormone production during pregnancy (or while on birth control pills) is the major contributor to this condition, which seems to be more prevalent in dark-haired, dark-skinned women. Sun exposure can heighten the discoloration, so always wear sunscreen. Treatment options include over-the-counter or prescription skin-bleaching products, light chemical peels, and laser resurfacing.

- ✔ **Moles:** Those little brown bumps are actually tumors of the skin's pigment-producing cells, but you don't need to panic — most moles develop in early childhood and are not a health threat. However, you must watch moles carefully because they can turn cancerous, and you should have a dermatologist immediately examine any new moles that appear. Because most people have at least 20 to 30 moles sprinkled around their bodies, regular skin checks are a must, especially in climates where large areas of skin are regularly exposed to strong sunlight.

The only way to remove a mole is to have it surgically removed; otherwise, it can grow back. See a dermatologist or a plastic surgeon.

✔ **Vitiligo:** A genetic condition of hypopigmentation, vitiligo occurs when melanin is absent in certain areas of the skin. On the face, you usually see the lack of pigment around the mouth and eyes. The depth of your natural skin tone determines how noticeable the condition is; use sunscreen diligently and avoid the sun to keep the problem from intensifying. Skin-bleaching agents such as hydroquinone can help promote a more even appearance in the skin; special-cover makeup products (such as Dermablend) are useful for unifying skin tone.

Dermatologist Patricia Wexler, M.D., says, "Vitiligo is a difficult problem. There are certain sun sensitizers you can use, and you can be given light therapy to actually attract the sun to try to stimulate the regrowth of the pigment. Some doctors use topical cortisone, and some actually give cortisone by mouth. In very extreme cases, it's easier to take away the rest of the color than it is to bring back color."

Skin cancer

Skin cancer is the most common form of cancer in the U.S. Left untreated, it can be fatal, but the good news is that it is almost entirely avoidable: Because 95 percent of skin cancers are caused by sun exposure, avoiding prolonged sun time and wearing a high-SPF sunscreen greatly decrease your risk. Caught early, most types of skin cancer can be successfully treated and eliminated, so get regular, thorough skin checks, especially if you have one or more of the following risk factors:

✔ Very fair skin that burns or blisters easily in the sun

✔ A close relative with skin cancer

✔ A history of prolonged sun exposure

✔ Two or more severe sunburns in your lifetime

✔ Moles that are unusual in appearance: uneven in shape, mixed in color, having irregular borders, or bigger than a pencil eraser

✔ An unusual number of moles (40 or more is considered beyond normal)

✔ Residence in a region with strong UV radiation, such as the southern United States or an area of high elevation

Dermatologist Patricia Wexler, M.D., says, "Because we're diagnosing skin cancer in people so young, ages 17 and up, I'm a big believer in a yearly professional checkup, either with an internist or family practitioner or with a dermatologist. Certainly people should be aware that if they were born with any spots that have hair within the mole, these are lesions that have a higher risk of changing. Any spots you have should be watched for change of color and shape, bleeding, crusting, or irregularity in the border. If anything grows rapidly or changes in color or shape, you should see a specialist."

Skin cancer tumors can be either benign (non-cancerous) or malignant (cancerous). Existing moles or birthmarks may become cancerous, or an entirely new mark, freckle, bump, or spot may be the first sign of a new tumor. If you see any suspicious changes in your skin, see a dermatologist immediately. With early detection and removal, doctors can successfully treat or cure most skin cancers. Treatment varies depending on the size and depth of the affected area. Often, basal and squamous cell carcinomas can be entirely eliminated when removed for biopsy. Other methods include laser removal, curettage (scraping the skin with a sharpened instrument), radiation therapy, topical chemicals, and cryosurgery (freezing).

Vascular irregularities

These skin flaws are tied to the body's veins and capillaries — part of your body's circulatory system — so no amount of AHA, pimple medication, or skin-bleaching cream can make them go away. You need a physician's involvement for correction.

- ✔ **Birthmarks:** Not to be confused with odd areas of brown-toned pigmentation caused by melanin, vascular birthmarks are typically red or reddish in hue. Vascular birthmarks are usually more of a nuisance than a health threat, but you should observe them carefully and report any changes to a dermatologist immediately. Laser correction is by far the most effective way to eliminate such marks; special-cover makeup is also useful, though temporary.

- ✔ **Rosacea:** Sometimes referred to as acne rosacea or adult acne, rosacea is a confusing skin problem because it resembles acne but is actually a disorder of the blood vessels. Rosacea is most common in fair-skinned women over 20 years of age, and is typified by facial ruddiness and red, pimple-like bumps on the cheeks and nose. Rosacea does not respond to typical acne medications — in fact, treating the skin with drying acne products often irritates it further — so a dermatologist's intervention is necessary. Although the root cause of rosacea is still unclear, its triggers are well known: stress, sunlight, extreme temperature changes, hot beverages, alcohol, spicy foods, hormonal changes, and pregnancy —

anything that causes the skin to flush. There's no cure for rosacea, but medications such as oral and topical antibiotics and steroids can help keep it in check.

✔ **Spider veins:** Usually caused by gravity and common in those who stand for long periods of time, these small, red veins can also result from pregnancy, hormonal imbalances, or genetic predisposition. Smoking, alcohol, and spicy diets also tend to promote their appearance, especially on the face, and they're often linked to acne rosacea. Treatment options include laser correction or electrocoagulation, which destroys the vessel by passing a low-voltage current through a needle. You can also camouflage spider veins with special-cover makeup like Dermablend.

Keeping Skin at Its Best

The past decade has seen some truly remarkable advances in skin care. And along with the new technology comes a new attitude: Instead of letting things slide until surgery must be done, the current approach is to correct small problems as they arise — which may just help you avoid the big ones altogether. So many safe, effective, non-invasive options for maintaining your skin's look are now available that, says dermatologist Joel Kassamir, M.D., "whether it's glycolic acids or Retin-A or Erbium lasers or collagen injections, there's a way to incorporate them all to give the patient a better look without picking up a scalpel."

Products

Until recently, any skin care product that claimed to counteract the visible signs of aging was highly suspect. Now, a few available ingredients really do have an impact on keeping skin smooth, healthy, and supple. This section talks about some of the most common skin-enhancing products.

Alpha and beta hydroxy acids

Alpha and beta hydroxy acids (AHAs and BHA) seem to be everywhere these days. These very popular ingredients help skin look smoother and fresher by speeding up its exfoliation rate. By chemically weakening the "glue" that holds spent cells to the skin's surface, they help new cells emerge more quickly and uniformly, resulting in smoother, clearer skin. "There's no doubt that these acids give your face a fresher look," says dermatologist Joel Kassamir, M.D. "They accelerate cell turnover and help clear the pores of debris or makeup." However, overuse can dry and irritate skin, and the positive effects last only as long as you continue to use products that contain these ingredients.

- ✔ **AHAs**, also known as fruit acids, are derived from sugar cane (glycolic acid), fruit (citric acid), apples (malic acid), milk (lactic acid), grapes (tartaric acid), and other substances. Glycolic acid is considered to have the best penetration capabilities and is the AHA that's most often used in chemical peels (described later in this chapter).

- ✔ **BHA** (salicylic acid) has been used in dermatology for decades to keep the skin clear. It penetrates more deeply into pores than AHAs, making it effective for anti-acne use. And because it's a derivative of aspirin (acetylsalicylic acid), it's also believed to contain similar anti-inflammatory properties.

Because of the craze for these ingredients — AHAs especially — they have been added to everything from facial cleansers to body lotions. For maximum effectiveness as exfoliants, AHAs need to be in a concentration of 5 percent or above, and BHA at a 1 to 2 percent level. However, *too* much is also a problem, as it can be highly irritating to the skin. The best way to be sure that you're getting a safe, appropriate AHA product is to ask your dermatologist or aesthetician for a recommendation.

Antioxidants

As their name says, antioxidants are in the business of thwarting oxidants — specifically free radicals, which are unstable molecules that "oxidize" and age the skin. Antioxidants such as vitamins A, C, and E, beta carotene, and selenium neutralize the free radicals that can damage the skin. They also may stimulate collagen and can help sunscreen agents work more effectively. Vitamin C in particular has been shown to improve superficially sun-damaged skin. No solid evidence has determined exactly how much antioxidant must be used, or whether it's effective at preventing skin damage over the long run. However, the consensus is that antioxidants do hold promise as anti-aging ingredients.

Bleaching creams

You used skin-lightening products to even out areas of hyperpigmentation on the skin, but these products don't actually *bleach* the skin. Their active ingredient — either hydroquinone or kojic acid — inhibits melanin production, so the skin can't produce darker pigment on the areas where you apply it. Results take several weeks to appear. Most drugstores carry a few different brands (sometimes referred to as "fade creams"), which typically contain 1 to 2 percent hydroquinone; prescription formulas have around 3 to 4 percent.

Using skin-bleaching products in conjunction with AHAs, BHA, and Retin-A aids their penetration and speeds the exfoliation of old, dark cells; your dermatologist can advise you on a good combination. You must wear sunscreen during and after use of these products, or hyperpigmentation returns.

Tretinoin

Tretinoin (you may know it by the trade name Retin-A) is a vitamin A derivative long used to treat acne. This potent exfoliant causes skin to shed its top layer within a few days of application. Used regularly, it prompts faster, more efficient cell turnover and has been shown to stimulate collagen production. Tretinoin has become hugely popular for its skin-renewing effects: diminishing the appearance of fine lines, preventing blemishes, keeping pores clear, smoothing the skin's texture, evening out irregular pigmentation, and promoting a healthy-looking glow. It may also help skin shed precancerous lesions.

This product has some negatives, too, including prolonged skin dryness, redness, and discomfort while your skin develops a tolerance to the product. It may prompt your skin to react to other skin care products. Ask your doctor to recommend a moisturizer to counteract irritation and peeling. Plus, tretinoin costs approximately $35 to $50 per tube, which some insurance plans may not cover.

Available only by prescription in the U.S., tretinoin comes in strengths from 0.25 percent to 1 percent and in gel and cream formulas. Results usually appear after a few months of regular use — which you must keep up if you want the results to last. Tretinoin sensitizes the skin to the sun, so tanning is out of the question, and daily use of a high-SPF sunscreen is a must.

Procedures

These non-invasive, non-surgical methods rejuvenate the look of the skin. Some of them can be done during your lunch hour, and no one will be the wiser. Others are considerably more involved — but you shouldn't enter into any of them lightly. Although a dermatologist can do most of these procedures in his or her office, plastic surgeons also perform some of them.

Because the physician's skill level makes all the difference in the results, you must be certain that the physician you choose is adept and experienced at the procedure you're requesting. See the "Finding a doctor" sidebar later in this chapter for tips on finding the right doctor for your needs.

Botox

Originally used to stop facial tics and spasms, Botox (produced from botulism toxin) temporarily paralyzes the muscles into which it's injected. Because facial contractions result in wrinkling or furrowing — especially on the forehead and around the eyes — Botox prevents you from making those faces, so the skin over the injection site stays smooth. Botox's effects gradually wear off in about four months, but, says dermatologist Fred Brandt, M.D., "because you've not been doing the muscle contractions which cause the lines during that time, even when the Botox wears away, the lines will not be as deep as they would have been if constant muscle contractions had been occurring, which is a great benefit."

Dermatologist Patricia Wexler, M.D., says, "Botox has revolutionized the treatment of the upper third of the face. Before, all these furrows and creases were treated with filling materials like collagen or silicone. But these lines are mechanical — they're due to expressions being made — so the minute you go home and squint, the lines come back. Botox actually treats the cause of the line; you're preventing the line from being there by paralyzing a muscle that you don't want to contract. And there's virtually no risk. People are afraid of Botox because it's called botulism, but the incidence of problems is under 5 percent for the general public and under 1 percent for people who use it constantly in their practice."

Best for: Frown lines between the eyes, crow's feet.

Pain factor: Minimal. A pinprick at the injection site, followed by a mild burning sensation that wears off in minutes.

Recovery time: Patients are encouraged to avoid lying down for a few hours to keep the solution from traveling to other areas of the face; the full effect of the injection takes about a week to develop.

Potential problems: Eyelid droop if injected too close to the eye; too-zealous injection at multiple sites on the face can hinder facial expression.

Cost: $300 to $500 per problem area.

Chemical peels

All chemical peels work in the same way: By creating a controlled inflammation of the skin's outer layers, they prompt the skin to shed — taking with it problems such as pigmentation irregularities and superficial wrinkles — and encourage the growth of fresh, smooth skin. Light, "lunch-hour" peels are a great way to keep skin clear and glowing; deeper peels, which have a rejuvenating effect on skin's collagen, leave skin more supple and elastic but also carry more risk and recovery time. Your skin may flake or peel a few days after the peel, but flaking or peeling usually subsides quickly.

"You're probably better off doing frequent light peels," says dermatologist Joel Kassamir, M.D. "You still accelerate cell turnover, but recuperation is trivial and the risk of developing scars or deep pigmentation is reduced." If deeper resurfacing is needed, a more modern approach is an Erbium laser. You can find more information about laser treatments later in this chapter.

Depending on your skin's needs, your dermatologist will choose one of the following three chemicals, arranged from a light peel to a more aggressive peel.

Stay out of the sun for at least two weeks after a chemical peel. If you're exposed to sun, a sever sunburn could result. As a general rule, if you receive regular chemical peels, you are more prone to sun damage, so be careful and protect your skin with sunscreen or by wearing a hat.

AHA peels

This light peel typically uses glycolic acid in concentrations of 30 to 70 percent to remove the outer layers of the epidermis. The solution is swabbed onto the skin, left on for a few minutes, and then rinsed off with water. Though most people tolerate glycolic acid well, many dermatologists prefer to perform AHA peels over a series of visits, gradually building up to higher concentrations to minimize any possible risk.

In the wrong hands, even a light AHA peel can be harmful, so never trust your skin to anyone but a qualified physician. "A patient of mine had a glycolic peel at a facialist," says dermatologist Fred Brandt, M.D. "They put it on her skin even though she'd been picking some pimples — and you can't put glycolic acid on damaged skin. It's taken up through that area much deeper than it would be on intact skin, so she got tons of scabbing and crusting. Fortunately, she was fine, but women need to realize that there are a lot of nuances to these peels. You can theoretically scar the skin with glycolic acid, so I feel that all these peels should be done at a doctor's office."

Best for: Eliminating fine lines, evening skin tone and texture, preventing and clearing up blemishes, restoring skin's glow.

Pain factor: Light stinging upon application that subsides after a few minutes.

Recovery time: One hour to two weeks for redness to subside from the strongest peels. Easily covered with makeup when allowed (usually a few hours after the procedure).

Potential problems: Sunburn-like reaction or discoloration; both are rare.

Cost: About $100 to $300 per session; a program of six sessions at one-month intervals is common. A one-time deep peel costs around $1,000.

Glycolic peels really helped my acne, and I think they're a great way for women with fine lines to help their skin look a little smoother. It's a 15-minute procedure — no surgery or anything heavy about it — and the healing time is virtually nothing. Whether you're doing it to reduce fine lines or to control acne, the result is the same — you leave the doctor's office with your skin *glowing.*

TCA (trichloroacetic acid) peels

Depending on the concentration used (from 10 to 70 percent), TCA can create a very mild or a very deep peeling effect on the skin. It's usually used for moderate-depth procedures that reach the top level of the dermis. The application procedure is similar to that for AHA peels, but TCA treatments usually take about a half-hour, and more passes or different strengths may be used on different parts of the face — lighter in the eye area, for example, where skin is thinner.

Best for: Eliminating deeper wrinkles or evening out marked pigmentation problems. Can also be used on the hands.

Pain factor: Mild to moderate, depending on the depth of the peel. Sedation is usually given for more aggressive procedures.

Recovery time: With lighter peels, skin becomes red and swollen. This effect subsides in three to seven days, and you can then wear makeup. With deeper peels, swelling and oozing occur afterward. The skin crusts over and peels in a week or two, revealing pink skin that you can cover with makeup. Normal skin tone returns a few weeks later.

Potential problems: Pigmentation loss, too-deep peeling; can activate cold sores or acne in those who are predisposed.

Cost: About $1,000 to $4,000, depending on the extent of the procedure.

Phenol peels

Phenol penetrates to the mid-level of the dermis, making it very effective on the deepest wrinkles and the most profound sun damage. However, phenol is also very invasive — the heart must be monitored during full-face procedures — so it's used very little today; lasers can do the same thing with less health risk. Application follows a swab-on procedure similar to AHAs and TCA, and the results are long-lasting. Because phenol peels can impair the skin's ability to tan, sun exposure is strictly forbidden post-procedure.

Best for: Resurfacing the deepest wrinkles and evening severe pigmentation problems; also useful for removing and preventing the recurrence of precancerous and cancerous lesions.

Pain factor: Phenol numbs the skin as it's applied, so pain during application is minimal (in addition, sedation is used). Post-procedure discomfort may require prescription painkillers.

Recovery time: 48 hours of post-procedure bed rest is recommended; some patients opt for hospitalization or home care. Skin is red, swollen, and oozy for eight to ten days until scabs form; the scabs slough off two to three weeks later. The fresh skin is pink to red but gradually fades to normal in three to six months.

Potential problems: Scarring, too-deep peeling, skin atrophy, marked loss of pigmentation; damage to heart, kidneys, and liver; can activate cold sores or acne in those who are predisposed. Not recommended for dark skin or diabetics.

Cost: $1,500 to $4,000, depending on the extent of the procedure.

Collagen injections

A temporary way to rejuvenate the skin's look, collagen injection utilizes bovine collagen (derived from cow skin) to plump up wrinkles and de-pressed scars. The collagen is injected by syringe into the areas to be treated; several areas of the face (forehead, cheeks, and smile lines) can be done in one session. The body breaks down injected collagen, so what's been added gradually "deflates" over a period of months. Just how quickly this occurs depends on what and how much was injected, but the results typically last four to six months.

Because bovine collagen can cause allergic reactions in some individuals, one or two pre-procedure skin tests are necessary to rule out any potential problems.

Best for: Filling in small facial creases and recessed scars; plumping up lips; smoothing frown and smile lines.

Pain factor: Mild — although some areas are more sensitive than others. A topical agent can be applied to lessen pain.

Recovery time: With skin, a few hours to a few days until spot-redness and tenderness subside. With lips, swelling and sensitivity last two to three days.

Potential problems: Allergic reaction to bovine collagen, too-fast reabsorp-tion into the body, possible link to autoimmune disorders. Bruising also may occur.

Cost: Depends on the amount injected; usually $300 to $1,000 per visit.

Dermabrasion

One of the longest-used skin-resurfacing procedures, dermabrasion uses a high-speed rotary wire brush or diamond disk to sand the top layer of skin cells from the face or body. Though it has fallen out of frequent use in favor of chemical peels and laser resurfacing, it's sometimes used in tandem with those procedures on areas that need extra help, such as the upper lip or cheeks. Spot procedures can take as little as a few minutes; full-face derm-abrasion can take up to an hour.

Best for: Evening out surface irregularities, especially deep wrinkles, acne scars, and pockmarks; smoothing vertical lip-area lines; and resurfacing heavy, thick skin.

Pain factor: None during the procedure because anesthetic is given. Afterward, moderate discomfort may call for painkillers.

Recovery time: Post-procedure, skin is raw, oozing, and red and usually is covered with a surgical dressing. Scabs form and then fall off in ten days to two weeks, exposing reddened skin that can be covered with makeup. Normal color returns in three to six months.

Potential problems: Scarring, infection, uneven results, pigment irregularities; can activate cold sores or acne in those who are predisposed. Not recommended for dark skin.

Cost: Depends on the amount of area covered and the number of sessions needed. Spot dermabrasion ranges from $200 to $900, whereas full-face dermabrasion costs much more.

Fat transplants

Fat injections are called *transplants* because they move living tissue from one body site to another. Using a syringe, your doctor takes fat from a donor site on your own body (usually the thighs or buttocks), prepares it, and then injects it into areas that need plumping. Your fat is then stored and can be used for up to a year. (Smile lines, pitted scars, and lips are common, but it can be used anywhere on the face and body.) Because your own tissue is being used, there's no chance of an allergic reaction, but fat's slightly thicker consistency keeps it from being injected as precisely as collagen.

Fat is a living substance, so its longevity once transplanted depends on its ability to link with the area's blood supply — an iffy process at best. Though some fat (typically 10 to 20 percent of each injection) *will* make that link and stay in place permanently, the other 80 to 90 percent dissipates in about six months. The same site may need to be reinjected several times until enough fat "takes" to give the desired result.

Best for: Moderate facial creases, skin depressions, and smile and frown lines; plumping the lips.

Pain factor when removing the fat: Tiny incisions are made for inserting the needle to remove the fat. Pain is minimal; the procedure usually is done without pain medication, although you can request it. Stitches are necessary where incisions are made. The physician tightly wraps the buttocks and thighs to avoid any indentations where the fat has been removed.

Pain factor when injecting the fat: The areas treated are not usually given any sort of anesthetic, although you can request a topical anesthetic; the discomfort is minimal.

Recovery time for removal of fat: Mild discomfort can last for one to two days, and deep bruising will probably occur.

Recovery time for injection of fat: Soreness and swelling in the injected areas can last for one to two days, and bruising is common.

Potential problems: Imprecise placement; rapid reabsorption requiring frequent touch-ups.

Cost: From about $800 to $5,000, depending on the extent of the treatment. (Check with your dermatologist for an accurate estimate of what this procedure costs in your area.)

Laser resurfacing

The new and very popular laser resurfacing works by simultaneously vaporizing the upper levels of the skin and tightening the collagen layer beneath. Very fast and accurate, the laser is computer-guided to release tiny bursts of light, removing the wrinkled skin to the necessary depth and leaving the underlying layer intact. The physician also treats some areas freehand, sometimes making several passes with the laser, wiping away vaporized skin between passes. Because laser resurfacing encourages collagen to reorganize itself in a smoother fashion, it's also an effective way to minimize raised scars. Extensive resurfacing is normally done in a hospital-type setting. A full-face laser resurfacing takes about an hour.

"I've been doing laser peels for about four years, and it's exciting to see the technology evolve," says dermatologist Patricia Wexler, M.D. "The carbon dioxide laser used to be used to get rid of wrinkles and tighten the skin, but in the past year, the Erbium laser has gotten very popular. Erbium is what I call 'laser lite'; it has a much quicker healing time. Most people who have Erbium laser treatments are back at work six or seven days after the procedure versus two weeks for the carbon dioxide laser, and any redness they have is almost always gone in one month versus three to six months. It's great for people with mild to moderate sun damage — and patients like it better because it's less painful, they heal quicker, and the redness is gone faster."

Misinformation given to patients has been the cause of dissatisfactory results from laser surgery. Laser resurfacing will not replace any type of face lifting, yet patients are sometimes told that a simple laser procedure will eliminate the need for forms of face lifting.

Best for: Eliminating superficial wrinkles, evening out pigmentation and skin texture, scar minimization and correction, spot resurfacing around the eyes and mouth.

Pain factor: Minimal. You may feel a slight snapping sensation, but anesthesia is usually given either locally for spot treatments or intravenously for full-face procedures. You may need painkillers for post-procedure discomfort.

Recovery time: Depends on the laser used and the depth of penetration. Light resurfacing can heal in a week or two; deeper work can leave the face red, swollen, and oozy for the first few days (a dressing is often applied). The skin crusts after about a week and then flakes off for another week, exposing new, red skin that fades to normal over a one- to four-month period. You can use makeup after the skin heals completely.

Potential problems: Scarring and irregular pigmentation, especially in darker skins; can activate cold sores or acne in those who are predisposed.

Cost: Depends on the area to be done. Spot scar-correction treatments can cost from $250; regional peels (such as the upper lip or eyes) cost $1,500 to $2,000; and full-face resurfacing ranges from $2,500 and higher.

Laser removal

Not to be confused with laser *resurfacing,* laser *removal* is concerned with pigmentation problems (such as age spots and tattoos) and vascular flaws (such as spider veins and birthmarks). The lasers work by emitting a wavelength of light that seeks a certain color in the skin. When it finds that color (red, for example), the laser's energy pulverizes it — without affecting the surrounding skin — and the fragments are swept away by the body's inner cleansing processes.

Best for: Broken capillaries, facial veins, birthmarks, scar improvement, and tattoo removal.

Pain factor: Mild to moderate. A local anesthetic can be given if extensive or sensitive areas are being treated.

Recovery time: Depends on the area treated and the type of laser used. Vascular removal lasers can leave the skin pink for a few hours; post-procedure bruising is common. With pigment removal lasers, some bleeding and blistering may occur. Skin heals with a crusted-over surface, which falls off in one to two weeks to reveal smooth, pink skin.

Potential problems: Incomplete removal of pigment; area may heal lighter, darker, or with a different texture than surrounding skin.

Cost: About $800 per session. You may need several sessions for total correction.

Finding a doctor

Any procedure you have done to your face is a major undertaking, so working with a skilled physician you can trust is crucial. With high demand for cutting-edge techniques such as laser resurfacing and chemical peels, some practitioners have jumped on the bandwagon without the necessary training and experience — and must be avoided at all costs. It's *your* responsibility to scrutinize any physician carefully to be sure that he or she is well-qualified in the techniques that you want. Here are a few tips for finding the right doctor for the job:

✔ **Compile a list of possible candidates.** Word-of-mouth really works here. Get referrals from friends and acquaintances who've had similar procedures, and from your family physician. For plastic surgery, you can call your local hospital(s) and ask for the names of board-certified plastic surgeons on staff; you can also call the ASPRS (American Society of Plastic and Reconstructive Surgeons) at 800-635-0635.

✔ **Check each candidate's credentials and affiliations.** For any surgical procedure, the doctor you choose must be board-certified in *plastic and reconstructive surgery.* Three trustworthy certifying bodies are the American Board of Plastic Surgery (ABPS), the American Society of Aesthetic Plastic Surgeons (ASAPS), and the American Association of Aesthetic Surgeons (AAAS). In addition to board certification, the doctor should belong to a reputable professional organization; ASPRS is one of the best-respected and allows you to call for information about its member physicians.

✔ **Check out the candidates in person.** Make an appointment with at least three physicians, and pay careful attention to all aspects of your consultation. How long are you left waiting in the reception area? Does the doctor listen to you carefully, encourage you to ask questions, and answer all your queries thoroughly? Does he or she discuss the risks of the procedure as well as the benefits? Is he or she candid about his or her experience and fees? Nix any doctor who seems arrogant, pushy, unsure, or too busy to give you his or her complete and respectful attention.

✔ **Check the candidates' training.** Ask the doctor how he or she was trained in the procedure and how many times he or she has done the procedure, and talk to patients who've had the procedure performed by that physician. If you're a woman of color, make sure that the doctor has experience doing the procedure with your ethnic type, because possible pigmentation changes are always a concern.

The most common mistake women make is to set their sights on whichever doctor is hot at the moment, whether the doctor was just written up in a magazine or because the doctor has a lineup of celebrity clients. Although high-profile doctors are no doubt well-qualified, they're not necessarily the best choice for *you.* Consider them as possible doctors for the job, put them through the same scrutiny as you do the other physicians on your list, and *then* make your decision.

Chapter 4

Skin Q & A

· ·

In This Chapter

▶ Helpful answers to your questions about skin

▶ Common skin problems explained — and solved

· ·

Skin troubles can range from the easily remedied — dark undereye circles caused by lack of sleep, for example — to difficult problems that require a doctor's attention. The next time the unexpected pops up, don't panic. This chapter can help you figure out what's going on with your skin and, if necessary, treat the problem accordingly.

What Do I Do When I'm Just Not Looking My Best?

If your skin just isn't looking its best, refer to Table 4-1 to discover some common problems — and solutions to those problems.

Table 4-1	Skin Problems and Solutions	
Problem	**Cause**	**Solution**
Undereye puffiness	Not enough sleep	Cold compresses; cooling eye gel
	Too much alcohol	Drink fluids to rehydrate the skin
Dark circles	Not enough sleep	Cold compresses; firming eye cream
	Heredity	Corrective makeup (see Chapter 14)
Undereye flaking	Dehydrated skin	Eye cream day and night; increase water intake; use a room humidifier
	Allergic reaction to eye-area products	Discontinue use of those products; if the problem persists, see a dermatologist
Blotchy, lifeless skin	Dehydration	Increase water intake

(continued)

Table 4-1 (continued)

Problem	Cause	Solution
Blotchy, lifeless skin	Smoking	Quit! (see Chapter 1)
	Slow skin cell turnover	Exfoliate regularly; have chemical peels done
Clogged pores	Improper makeup removal/facial cleansing	Remove makeup and cleanse skin thoroughly; exfoliate regularly
	Oil-containing products	Switch to oil-free products
	Acne	Switch to an oily skin regimen (see Chapter 2); if the problem persists, see a dermatologist
Breakouts	Clogged pores (see above); diet (see Chapter 1)	Topical over-the-counter medication; prescription oral and/or topical antibiotics from a dermatologist
	Birth control pill/hormones	See an obstetrician/gynecologist

If I'm Breaking Out, Should I Exfoliate My Skin?

If you're prone to red pimples that are inflamed, using a calming mask may be better than exfoliating by rubbing the skin. Consider using a clay mask, which draws blackheads out of the skin in a non-aggressive manner by dehydrating the top layer of skin and pushing blackheads out.

I've Heard That the Rays from a Tanning Bed Can Help Clear Up Acne. Is This True?

Most dermatologists consider any type of tanning to be detrimental to the skin, although some people who suffer from acne feel that a slight tan lessens its appearance. Dermatologists don't prescribe sunlight for treatment of acne because the sun actually damages the skin and can cause wrinkles, malignant spots, and actual malignant skin cancers. In fact, sunlight or tanning bed exposure can induce new acne bumps.

Can Birth Control Pills Cause Breakouts?

Oral contraceptives can either clear up or cause acne, depending on their formulation. Because oral contraceptives contain androgen-like substances (the male hormone that can set off acne), they may make acne worse. However, many oral contraceptives actually improve acne. If you develop pimples after you begin taking oral contraceptives, ask your doctor about switching to another formula.

What Can I Do about My Acne Scars?

It's not too late to help your scarring. Today, several options are available for resurfacing your scars, the most popular being skin resurfacing and collagen injections. Although none of these procedures can return your skin to its pre-acne condition, they can help level out scars and give the skin a better overall appearance. See a dermatologist to learn more about your options.

What Should I Do When I Have an Adverse Reaction to Something?

Everyone's skin reacts differently to ingredients in skin care and cosmetic products. If your skin acts up after you use a product, you're likely seeing either an irritant reaction or an allergy. An irritant reaction appears right away and generally disappears after you stop using the product containing the offending ingredient. However, an allergic reaction, which occurs when the body recognizes part of a product's formula as a foreign substance, can be harder to shake and may require a doctor's visit. It's even possible to suddenly develop an allergic reaction to a product that you've used for years. You may discover that a manufacturer has changed the ingredients in a skin care product, cosmetic product, deodorant, or perfume that you've used for years, causing you to have an allergic reaction. If you think that you've experienced an allergic reaction, stop using the product immediately. If the irritation persists for more than a week, see a dermatologist.

To avoid adverse reactions, test a new skin care or cosmetic product on a small area before you buy it. Ask for a sample and try the product for a few days; you'll notice any irritant reaction immediately.

Common skin irritants

Women with dry skin should avoid the following ingredients:

- **Acetone:** Removes oil from the skin surface.

- **Alpha-hydroxy acids (AHAs):** Mild acids derived from fruits and other natural substances. May cause irritation, especially if used on the delicate skin around the eyes.

- **Alcohol:** Very drying. Look for alcohol esters and cetyl alcohol, which don't have alcohol's irritating effect.

- **Benzoyl peroxide:** A disinfectant and drying agent that's often used to treat acne. Can be very irritating to dry skin.

- **Camphor:** Found in many acne products.

- **Citrus juices:** High acid content can irritate the skin.

- **Eucalyptus:** A potential irritant found in acne products.

- **Menthol:** Can be irritating.

- **Mint:** Can feel cool and refreshing, but may irritate the skin on the face.

- **Salicylic acid:** A beta-hydroxy acid and mild exfoliant that can irritate the skin.

Women with oily skin need to watch out for oils in skin care products, including

- **Alcohol:** May be too drying, except for those with very oily skin.

- **Lanolin:** A common ingredient in moisturizers. May be too heavy for women with oily skin, and should be avoided by those with a history of eczema. Other forms of lanolin include lanolin alcohol, lanolin oil, acetylated lanolin, and hydroxylated lanolin.

- **Petroleum-based oils (mineral oil and petroleum jelly, for example):** Tend to leave a greasy film.

For years, whenever my skin broke out after I used a particular facial mask or cleanser, well-meaning facialists tried to convince me that my skin was simply purging "toxins." I no longer believe that argument. If a skin care product makes your skin break out, sting, swell, or redden, return it to the store and buy something else.

I Have Blackheads around My Nose. Will a Tape (Such as Biore Pore Perfect Strips) Help Me?

A tape may help remove your blackheads, but be careful if your skin is sensitive or dry. These tapes are effective on some people, but on others they can be ineffective as well as drying. It's better to use them on occasion than as a part of your daily skin care routine.

Because Sunlight Is a Source of Vitamin D, Isn't Avoiding the Sun Completely Actually Bad for You?

That's true — partly. Your skin needs some exposure to the sun in order to produce vitamin D. However, your skin gets enough sun exposure through daily activities, such as going to work or picking up the kids from school. There's no need to lie out in the sun to soak up vitamin D.

What's the Best Treatment for a Sunburn?

First of all, you should never get a sunburn if you use an SPF lotion, cover yourself, and take sensible precautions. However, if you do get burned, take aspirin as quickly as possible to help keep the inflammation down. Constantly apply fresh aloe vera gel or a cream suited for burns for the first 24 to 48 hours until the redness and stinging subside.

A first-degree sunburn causes redness of the skin and heals over a few days after you shed the upper layer of the epidermis. Topical and internal cortisones can help reduce the stinging and redness. A second-degree sunburn results in blisters and should be treated by a doctor, because you may experience fluid loss and even shock. Treatment includes steroids, both topical and internal, as well as cool soaks, antibiotics, and sometimes even tetanus re-immunization.

Should I Use Soap to Dry My Oily Skin?

No, you shouldn't use soap to try to dry out oily skin, says dermatologist Patricia Wexler, M.D. "It's the worst thing you can do, because when you have a lot of oil in your skin, using a topical astringent or soap dries the top layer of skin. The glands, which are deeper, think that the skin is dry and push out more oil, so you actually create a vicious cycle of stripping and then re-creating oils," she says.

Wexler points out that many companies are now making topical moisturizers that actually absorb oil from the surface of the skin. "Rather than trying to strip the skin of the oil, the oil is just sort of absorbed by this makeup as it's being released, and it's much healthier and more natural for the skin," she says. "Skin has a normal pH, and you shouldn't do so much to try to disrupt it, because if you strip the skin, you just have to reconstitute it. It's much better to use products that work within the normal function of the skin and that aren't too drying."

I Have Bluish Circles Under My Eyes, Even When I Get Enough Sleep. Why Is This?

The discoloration may be caused by veins that are visible through the very thin skin under your eyes. People with deep-set eyes tend to have blue circles. To lesson their appearance, always use eye cream to smooth out the skin's texture, followed by concealer, taking care to be very delicate with that fragile undereye skin.

Now That I'm in My Thirties, I See Little Brown Spots on My Face. Should I Be Concerned?

Those brown spots are likely caused by sun exposure, birth control pills, or pregnancy. They typically begin to appear in your thirties. You may be a candidate for reparative work, such as a Retin-A derivative, vitamin C, alpha-hydroxy acid, or even peels or laser surgery. A dermatologist can examine your skin and recommend an option.

I Want My Skin to Have a Healthy Glow. What Can I Do?

First, take good care of yourself by drinking water, eating well, and sleeping enough. Then follow this simple skin care regimen: gentle cleanser, moisturizer, sunscreen, and, most important, regular exfoliation. Exfoliating can mean using a washcloth, applying a cream that contains glycolic acid or salicylic acid, or having glycolic or acid peels. Exfoliation gives skin a fresh glow and eliminates patchy spots that make skin look blotchy or irregular.

My Pores Are Enormous. Is It Possible to Minimize Their Appearance?

You can minimize the appearance of large pores with the help of topical agents or medications prescribed by a dermatologist. Because oiliness can attract attention to areas of skin with large pores, keep your skin clean and minimize the shine on your skin with powder.

What's the Best Way to Deal with a Cold Sore?

Cold sores (also known as canker sores or fever blisters) are tiny, clear fluid-filled blisters caused by the herpes simplex virus. The type I virus usually is associated with infections on the face. Once you get the virus, it never leaves. Many people have only one active infection, and others see cold sores reappear every few weeks or months.

To treat a cold sore, rest and apply ice if the numbing soothes the pain. Because the herpes virus may be spread through kissing or directly touching the active sore, leave the area alone. Don't go out in the sun without extra protection (apply a lip balm containing SPF 15 or higher prior to sun exposure and reapply it every half-hour), and see a doctor if the cold sore lasts longer than two weeks.

Dermatologist Patricia Wexler, M.D., recommends the following cold sore treatment to her patients: "If they get cold sores infrequently, I tell them that the minute they feel the symptoms coming on, they should be taking a pill, like Valtrex or Doparax, which will stop the cold sore from coming on full-blown and may even prevent it from coming out if they catch it early enough. People who get recurring cold sores can be on a constant low maintenance of Valtrex or Doparax. There's no reason to suffer. These pills have almost no side effects and can be taken for months or years at a time." See a dermatologist for more information about these medications.

The herbal remedy for cold sores is Lyfine. It comes in ointment and pill forms and can be purchases at drugstores and health-food stores.

Part II

Hair

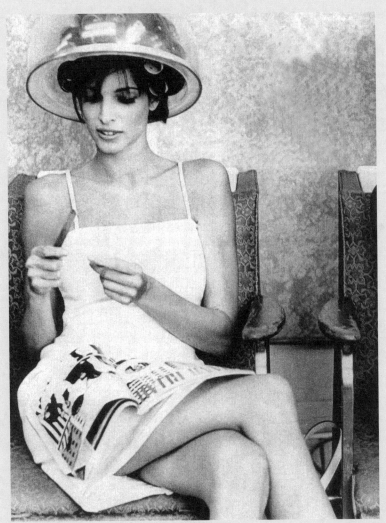

Pamela Hanson

In this part . . .

The human obsession with hair is age-old and well-documented. In ancient Greece, both men and women powdered their hair with pollen and gold dust to achieve a "blonde" effect; the Assyrians even enacted laws delineating the hairstyles that citizens could wear based on their social status. In this century, women have been bobbed, crimped, feathered, bouffant-ed, and pixied. Nothing else on your person can be changed so totally — or make you look so totally different when changed.

This part gets to the root of hair issues, from the products that really enhance hair's appearance, to finding your best cut and color, to pro tips for styling your hair at home.

Chapter 5

Hair Care Basics

. . . .

In This Chapter

▶ Shampoo and conditioner formulas and ingredients explained

▶ Cleansing and conditioning hair properly

▶ Understanding the difference between drugstore and salon products

. . . .

*T*he first and most important thing that you must know about your hair is how to care for it. Even if your hair has never been colored or processed, you still have to take certain measures to keep it in good condition. The key is to treat your hair as you treat your skin: Cleanse it gently, moisturize (condition) it when needed, and give it occasional extra pampering to keep it looking its best.

Hair care doesn't have to be complicated, and with so many shampoos and conditioners on the market, you're sure to find products that are right for you. And when you have the right products, you can do almost anything with your hair.

Shampoo Formulas

The main function of shampoo is to remove the sebum that the scalp naturally secretes, as well as to remove residual conditioning and styling products. The word *shampoo* itself is derived from the Hindu word *champo,* which means "to massage" or "to knead," reflecting the physical action that you use on the head. The first modern commercial shampoos were created in the 1930s by John Breck, whose obsession with his own thinning hair led him to formulate what would become the first mass-market hair care products in the world.

At heart, shampoos are pretty straightforward: water combined with a detergent or surfactant. The rest of the bottle is taken up by thickeners, detanglers, fragrance, and preservatives. These additional ingredients are what really make the difference between formulas. Table 5-1 compares the different shampoo formulas.

Table 5-1		Shampoo Formulas	
Type	*Point of Difference*	*Positives*	*Negatives*
Baby shampoo	Contains no eye-stinging ingredients	Great for babies, kids, and sensitive eyes	No conditioning properties; may not be strong enough for adults
"Blue" shampoo	Contains blue or violet pigments; specifically made for gray hair	Counteracts yellow cast common in gray hair	Limited selection of formulas
Clarifying shampoo	Contains few or no conditioning agents	Great for very oily hair and for removing product build-up	No conditioning properties; can strip away needed oils; too harsh for daily use by most hair types
Color-added shampoo	Contains dyes to enhance hair color	Can slightly enrich hair color and/or prolong the look of color-treated hair; adds sheen	Not effective for lasting color coverage
Conditioning shampoo	Contains conditioner	Great for overnight trips if you don't want to carry both shampoo and conditioner; good for kids or men who don't want two steps in the shower	Does not moisturize hair the way a separate conditioner does
Dandruff shampoo	Contains FDA-regulated ingredients proven to relieve dandruff	Helps control dandruff itching and recurrence	Can be harsh on hair and have a strong, unpleasant odor
Dry shampoo	Powder-form product that works without water	Freshens hair quickly; preserves existing style	Not a good choice for daily cleansing
Moisturizing shampoo	Cleanses without drying; contains ingredients that replenish hair's moisture	Good for daily use by most hair types	Can eventually leave residue on hair; not appropriate for oily scalps

Type	Point of Difference	Positives	Negatives
Oily hair shampoo	Specially formulated for oily hair; dries excess oil at the scalp	Gives weighed-down, oily hair a fluffier, more normal appearance	Can be drying
Volumizing shampoo	Few or no conditioning properties; contains water-attracting ingredients to swell the hair shaft	Boosts thickness and doesn't weigh down hair	Won't give you the volume that a thickening spray used with a hair-dryer will

Conditioner Formulas

The basic function of conditioner is to coat the hair shaft with ingredients that temporarily "patch" damaged areas of the cuticle, seal in needed moisture, and help protect against further harm. Conditioner also helps eliminate tangles, tame frizzies and flyaways, improve manageability, and boost shine. However, these effects are only temporary; the next time you shampoo, most of that coating goes right down the drain, so you have to reapply. That's because once hair is damaged, it stays damaged. Conditioner cannot "heal" the hair shaft; it can only help temporarily smooth a damaged cuticle and give hair the *appearance* of health — until it washes out.

As with shampoo, conditioners have a common base formula: water and *emollients* (a fancy word for oils). The ratio of these ingredients to water determines how "intensive" the conditioner is. Table 5-2 gives you the details about daily conditioning products; read on in this section for more information about deep-conditioning packs and other conditioning treatments.

Table 5-2	Daily Conditioner Formulas		
Type	**Point of Difference**	**Positives**	**Negatives**
Finishing rinse	Lightweight, very liquid formula	Detangles and conditions without weighing hair down; good for unprocessed hair and fine, limp hair	Not intensive enough for serious damage

(continued)

Table 5-2 *(continued)*

Type	Point of Difference	Positives	Negatives
Instant conditioner	Light to intense conditioning properties	Widest selection; restores a healthy look and protects against further damage; best for normal to damaged hair	Can weigh down fine hair and leave build-up if overused
Conditioner for chemically treated or severely damaged hair	Intense conditioning for hair that's been damaged by chemical processes	Smoothes the cuticle; leaves hair soft and shiny	If used daily, eventually weighs down the hair
Leave-in conditioner	Left on the hair, not rinsed out	Light to medium conditioning properties; helps ease styling; protects hair against heat and styling damage	Can weigh down hair and leave build-up; easy to overuse
Color-added conditioner	Contains dyes to enhance hair color	Can slightly enhance hair color and/or extend the look of color-treated hair	Doesn't give lasting color coverage; applying to roots can make hair limp
Acidic rinse	Mildly acidic pH works to close the cuticle of the hair, improving smoothness and shine; typical ingredients include vinegar and citrus extracts	Helps give hair more manageability and shine	Does not work as a conditioning agent
Detangler	Very lightweight liquid or lotion that is sometimes found in spray form	Great for fine or healthy hair that needs help only with comb-through and needs no real conditioning properties; gives hair more manage-ability and shine	Adds a step outside the shower to your hair care routine

Extra helps defined

Although shampoo and conditioner clearly perform different functions, you'll find that their labels have in common many of the ingredients in this list:

- **AHAs:** These popular skin-exfoliating ingredients have found their way into shampoos. At lower concentrations, AHAs can bind water to the hair, which adds moisture, while higher concentrations help deflake the scalp.

- **Amino acids:** Because amino acids are the smaller building blocks of proteins, the theory is that they should be able to make their way more easily into damaged areas of the cuticle. However, there's no evidence that this is actually the case, nor that amino acids have the same cuticle-protecting effect on the hair that larger-moleculed proteins have.

- **Botanicals:** Naturally derived oils and aqueous extracts of plants like rosemary, peppermint, and sage are popular because they often replace manufactured additives. They're usually included in such small amounts that their effect is negligible, but they can add a nice fragrance to a product.

- **Conditioners and emollients:** Included in this group are vegetable oils, mineral oil, lanolin, silicone derivatives, and fatty alcohols. (Don't let the word *alcohol* disturb you — cetyl, stearyl, lauryl, and myristyl alcohols are gentle and creamy, and also help thicken a formula.) These ingredients leave a protective coating on the hair, helping to smooth the cuticle, seal in moisture, and enhance shine. Too much, however, is a bad thing: Lanolin, mineral oil, and silicones in particular can leave the hair greasy and flat if used in too high a concentration.

- **Humectants:** Ingredients like glycerine and glycols (propylene and butylene) help attract water to the hair to keep it feeling moisturized.

- **Panthenol (vitamin B_5 derivative):** The only vitamin shown to have the capability to penetrate the hair shaft, panthenol works like most other conditioning ingredients, helping to boost hair's luster and moisture-retaining abilities.

- **Protein (including collagen and elastin):** Because the hair is made of the protein keratin, adding proteins to hair care products makes sense. They cling to the hair shaft and can penetrate slightly, helping hair feel thicker and giving the cuticle some protection against further damage.

- **Quaternary ammonium compounds:** These ingredients are widely used in shampoos and conditioners to help detangle the hair.

- **SPF:** Many hair care companies are adding sunscreen to their products. However, sun care products for hair are not tested by the same methods as those for skin, so they're not rated by the familiar numerical method. Although no one disputes that the sun can have a damaging effect on the hair, it's still not certain whether an SPF on the hair can completely protect it. For maximum protection, a hat or scarf is still your best bet.

When hair is feeling especially dry or has lost its sheen, a deep-conditioning treatment is the way to go.

- ✔ **Protein packs**, also known as deep conditioners or intense conditioning packs, are pretty much identical to daily conditioners in their ingredients, but their consistency is thicker and their conditioning properties are more intense. They are meant to be left in the hair longer than daily conditioners; many are heat-activated, which allows the hair shaft to open up and absorb moisture.

- ✔ **Hair masks** are similar to protein packs, the difference being that many hair masks include clay and/or minerals. These are good for boosting the health of oily hair because clay draws out moisture. Women with light-colored hair should opt for a different type of deep-conditioning treatment because the minerals that hair masks contain (copper in particular) can leave a residual tinge.

- ✔ **Hot oil treatments** are just that: mixtures of different oils (plant, animal, or silicone), typically combined with conditioning ingredients like panthenol and proteins, that help seal in moisture and add softness to the hair.

You can find deep-conditioning treatments wherever hair care products are sold, usually in single-use foil packets or plastic tubes.

Finding a Hair Care Routine for You

Rather than going through all the trial-and-error of finding exactly what works for you, read through Table 5-3 to find out what to do daily, weekly, and monthly based on your hair type and texture. If you have combination hair — for example, oily and curly — combine the advice for those two types.

Table 5-3		Hair Care Routines by Hair Type		
Type	**Definition**	**Daily**	**Weekly**	**Monthly**
Normal	Not oily, not dry; not too thick or thin; not chemically processed	Moisturizing shampoo followed by a finishing rinse if needed	Follow monthly routine weekly if you spend a lot of time in the sun or swim in salt-water or chlorinated pools	Clarifying shampoo and a protein pack left on for 10 to 15 minutes

Type	Definition	Daily	Weekly	Monthly
Oily	Scalp secretes too much oil; hair looks greasy at the roots	Oily hair shampoo, concentrated on the scalp; choose a conditioner formula based on what the rest of your hair needs, keeping conditioner away from the scalp and using it on alternating days	Clarifying shampoo	Use a protein pack or hair mask followed by your clarifying shampoo if the ends of your hair are dry and need extra moisture
Dry	Hair may feel brittle, frizzy, or flyaway; lacks sheen	Moisturizing shampoo and an instant conditioner; use leave-in conditioner on ends if needed	Leave instant conditioner on hair for more than five minutes if possible	Clarifying shampoo and a protein pack or hot oil treatment
Fine/Limp	Extremely straight, not a lot of mass, flat to the head	Volumizing shampoo followed on alternating days by a finishing rinse or instant conditioner, only on the ends	Clarifying shampoo	Try having hair colored profes- sionally to add volume
Coarse	Not smooth, bumpy texture, normally thick; similar in feeling to horse hair	Moisturizing shampoo and an instant conditioner	Clarifying shampoo followed by a heavier conditioner for chemically treated hair or a protein pack	Protein pack or hot oil treatment left on for as long as possible

(continued)

Table 5-3 *(continued)*

Type	Definition	Daily	Weekly	Monthly
Chemically treated	Hair that's been colored, permed, or chemically straightened	Moisturizing shampoo and a conditioner formulated for chemically treated or severely damaged hair; be careful with sun exposure, which only further damages your hair	Clarifying shampoo; leave instant conditioner on hair for 15 minutes	Protein pack made for chemically treated or severely damaged hair; leave on as long as possible

Shopping for Hair Care Products

I buy my hair care products at all kinds of places: at the drugstore, at the salon, at the beauty supply store. Spending a lot of money on your products is certainly easy to do, but I don't think that it's really necessary. I've been very happy with the way some inexpensive products have made my hair look. It's really about trying different things and seeing whether they give your hair what it needs to look its best.

Here are some tips to keep in mind while shopping:

- Because shampoos are in the business of *removing* stuff from the hair and conditioners are about *adding* to the hair shaft, you usually see more payoff from having extras such as color enhancers, proteins, and deep-conditioning properties in your conditioner.

- Because hair care products are considered cosmetics by the FDA, they are not closely scrutinized for language unless they make truly outrageous or medical-type claims (such as "Regrows Hair in Seven Days!"). Stick to products about which the language sounds realistic and to the point.

- If you like what they used to wash or condition your hair at the salon, ask if you can get those products at the local beauty supply store, where products tend to cost less.

- Don't be afraid to cross-shop. If an inexpensive shampoo from Company A works with the ultra-pricey conditioner from Company B, so be it.

- When buying individual conditioning packets, consider how much hair you have on your head. Longer hair usually needs more than one packet. Disposable plastic shower caps, which you can usually find in drugstores, are great for intensifying these treatments.

Caring for Your Hair

Shampoo and conditioner are the basic one-two for keeping hair in good shape. After you figure out which formulas are right for your particular hair needs, you're ready to discover how to use them to the best effect.

I've learned a few tricks that have really made a difference in my hair. First, I've found that alternating shampoo and conditioner helps my hair look its best, because when I use the same products all the time — even after just one bottle — I notice that my hair doesn't respond as well. I keep two products that I really like right in the shower and switch back and forth. Occasionally, I try something new, following the recommendations for my hair type.

When my hair starts to look dull and lifeless, I know that it's time to use a clarifying shampoo. They cleanse hair of all the goop that can weigh it down — the residues from overconditioning and the build-up from styling products that my normal shampoo just isn't getting out. I always keep a clarifying shampoo in my shower so that I remember to use it every month or so — especially after a shoot for which very heavy products were applied to my hair. I wash my hair with a clarifier and then follow it with a good conditioner. Afterward, I really do see a difference: My hair seems to have more body and shine.

Shampooing

Shampooing is essential to every woman's hair care routine, regardless of her hair type or texture. The most important thing to remember while shampooing your hair is to focus your efforts on the scalp. Follow these steps for the perfect shampooing technique:

1. **Wet hair thoroughly, allowing the water to smooth your hair straight down toward the back of your head.**

   The water should be comfortably warm, not hot — hot water can irritate and dry the scalp.

2. **Pour shampoo into the palm of one hand and then rub both palms together to evenly distribute the product.**

   Don't pour shampoo directly onto your head; you'll use way too much and have difficulty spreading it.

3. **Apply the shampoo to the top of your head and use your fingertips to massage it onto your scalp.**

   Don't worry about the rest of your hair; it will be cleansed as you rinse out the shampoo. Depending on your hair's thickness and length, you may need to repeat Steps 2 and 3 to get enough shampoo into your hair.

4. Rinse all the lather from your hair with plenty of warm, clean water.

Lift the hair gently at the roots with your fingertips to let the water get right down to your scalp. Let the water smooth your hair away from your face and down your back to keep it tangle-free. Continue rinsing until the water falling from your hair is completely clean.

Shampooing tipsheet

✔ Don't be afraid to wash your hair every day. Washing doesn't make hair fall out more, and it doesn't make it drier.

✔ If you have long hair, briefly brush your hair before washing to remove any loose, dead strands. You'll have less hair in your drain, and less chance of ratty tangles later.

✔ You do not have to lather, rinse, and repeat unless you have some sort of product or residue in your hair that calls for extra cleansing.

✔ Rinsing thoroughly is the most important step in shampooing your hair. If you do not rinse thoroughly, your hair will look dirty, dull, and heavy. If, after being rinsed extremely well, your hair still looks dirty, change shampoos and use a clarifying shampoo to clear off excess residue.

✔ Regular soap is not a good substitute for shampoo; it strips your hair and leaves a residue behind.

✔ You may need to change your shampoo seasonally. In summer, the scalp tends to produce more oil, so you may need to step up to a more cleansing formula. Wintertime's dryness may call for a gentle, conditioning shampoo.

✔ Dandruff shampoos can be very hard on the hair — especially if the hair is chemically processed — so use them only when needed.

✔ Color-added shampoos (and conditioners) can stain your tub, grout, shower curtain, towels — even your skin and fingernails. Immediately rinse splatters and extra product off anything that isn't hair.

✔ Save any shampoos that you don't like and use them to hand-wash your lacy underthings.

Conditioning

Most hair needs the extra care that conditioner provides, especially if it's exposed to heat-styling and chemical processing. Conditioning is the flip side of shampooing — you concentrate your efforts on hair's ends, where your hair needs the most moisture. Avoid conditioning the roots, especially if you have oily hair; the scalp's natural oil takes care of things up top.

1. **After shampooing, gently squeeze the excess water from your hair with your hands.**

2. **Place conditioner in your hand, rub your palms together to distribute the product evenly, and then work it into your hair *from the ends up.***

   Do not pour conditioner on top of your head and then rub it in; instead, focus on the ends, where your hair tends to be drier and more damaged.

3. **If you have long hair, gently comb through the ends with a wide-tooth comb to make sure that the conditioner is evenly distributed and to remove any tangles.**

4. **Rinse hair well, gently lifting sections of the hair to ensure that water can move freely throughout.**

   Let the water direct your hair so that it falls down your back.

5. **Gently squeeze the water from your hair with your hands, and then wrap your head in a towel to absorb excess moisture.**

   Do not rub vigorously with the towel; use it to gently squeeze out moisture.

Use these same steps for applying deep-conditioning treatments, but adjust the amount of time you leave in the deep conditioner according to your hair's needs.

Conditioner tipsheet

✔ Not sure how much conditioner to use? Go by the length of your hair. If it's less than 6 inches long, use just a silver dollar-sized dollop. If you have very long hair, you may need a handful of conditioner.

✔ The most important thing to remember with conditioner: You can definitely get too much of a good thing. If you overapply or use too heavy a formula, you'll end up greasy and flat instead of full-bodied. The best approach: See how *little* you can use and still get good results.

✔ If your hair's ends are very damaged or your hair is static-prone, you may need more than one conditioner. Keep a good daily-use product on hand for your everyday needs and complement it with a leave-in conditioner.

✔ To keep your color looking fresh, alternate your regular conditioner with a color-added conditioner once a week.

✔ You may not need to use conditioner every day if your hair's very short, very straight and fine, very oily, or very healthy. All hair can benefit from a light conditioner, but give your hair a break on some days.

✔ Shampoo and condition your hair first in the shower. That way, you can leave conditioner on your hair while you do everything else, giving it more time to absorb into the hair shaft.

✔ Be sure to thoroughly rinse conditioner from your hair. Excess residue on the hair shaft dulls shine and makes hair look dirty faster.

✔ Your hair can't get "used to" a conditioner; it can, however, develop a layer of conditioner build-up. If you normally use a conditioning shampoo, it may not be removing residues thoroughly — and may leave some residue of its own — so be sure to alternate it with a non-conditioning shampoo, or occasionally use a clarifying shampoo to keep build-up at bay and conditioner working its best.

✔ Want your hair to look extra shiny? Take a tip from hairstylist Frederic Fekkai: After you rinse out your conditioner, try a final rinse with cold water or an acidic finishing rinse. Both methods close the hair's cuticle, helping it lie down smoothly and reflect light more evenly.

Deep conditioner tipsheet

✔ **Use heat to boost the conditioner's effect.** You can do so in several ways: You can cover your hair with a plastic cap or bag while you lounge in the bath. You can wrap your head in a towel to retain your own body heat (if possible, warm the towel in the dryer first). You can use a hood attachment with your blow-dryer, or a heated cap made expressly for the purpose (found in larger drugstores and beauty supply stores). Whatever method you choose, here's the payoff: Because heat opens the hair's cuticle, more conditioner will be absorbed.

✔ **Use deep conditioner only when and where needed.** Unless your hair is severely dry or damaged, using a rich, heat-activated conditioner once a week is probably too much. Instead of bouncy, shiny locks, you'll get limp, weighed-down hair. As with your normal conditioner, make sure that you avoid the roots and concentrate on your hair's ends, especially if your scalp is oily.

✔ **Time it right.** You don't need to sleep overnight with your conditioner-filled hair under a shower cap. Twenty minutes is a good starting point for most hair needs; go a little more or less after checking your results.

✔ **Keep the conditioner off your forehead if you have acne-prone skin.** The emollients in the conditioner can cause breakouts.

✔ **While you have deep conditioner on your hair, use the time to take a bath, tweeze your eyebrows, or do your nails.** Or, next time you go to the salon for a manicure or pedicure, ask if you can sit under the dryer for 30 minutes with conditioner on your hair. It's a great way to get a lot accomplished in little time.

Cuticle care

The *cuticle* is hair's outermost layer, which covers and protects the layers beneath. Excessive heat styling and chemical processing can damage the cuticle and leave hair overly porous and dull.

Sometimes, though, a little bit of cuticle abuse is okay . . . a *little.* In the case of hair color, chemicals "lift" the cuticle to allow pigment into the hair shaft; this "fluffing" of the cuticle can help hair look thicker and fuller. Backcombing (otherwise known as *teasing*) also roughs up the cuticle, which is why it's an effective method for giving hair lift (only once in a blue moon, and gently). Just remember: The more you disturb the cuticle, the more you risk damaging your hair. Here are some simple tips for keeping the daily abuse to a minimum:

- ✔ **Treat wet hair with care.** When hair's wet, it's in its most vulnerable state, so cuticle-roughing maneuvers like rubbing, scrubbing, wringing, and brushing are all no-nos. *Gently* work shampoo into the hair, *gently* press out water with a towel, and *gently* detangle with a wide-tooth comb.

- ✔ **Minimize heat-styling.** Overzealous use of blow-dryers, curling irons, and pressing irons can fry the cuticle. Never leave high heat on one area of the hair for more than a few seconds, and give your hair a break as often as possible. Try letting your hair air-dry, followed by a few quick minutes of heat-styling to finish, instead.

- ✔ **Don't overmanipulate hair.** Anytime you create friction on and among the hair shafts by brushing, blow-drying, or even taking a long ride in a convertible, you harm the cuticle. Despite what Grandma told you, 100 strokes a night is not a good idea.

Chapter 6

Finding Your Style

*1*f you're like most women, you have an idea of what you want your hair to look like. You get ideas when you look at magazines or watch movies — for example, when you see Katharine Ross in *The Graduate* and love her hair, you're identifying with long hair. When you see Ava Gardner in *Night of the Iguana,* you know that you're identifying with something shorter and sexier. Or if you see Linda Evangelista on the cover of *Bazaar* with a short, sleek bob, you know that you're identifying with something modern and edgy.

Once you have a picture in your mind of your dream hairstyle, you have to adapt it to your hair type and face shape. For example, you may love Grace Kelly's hairstyle and cut, but you're a brunette and you know that you look best as a brunette. That's okay. Go with that hairstyle and your own hair color. Sometimes you have to be realistic and accept your hair's limitations. You may want Andie MacDowell's big, curly locks, but no matter how great your perm is, it's never going to look as beautiful as Andie's naturally curly hair. Finding a hairstyle that suits your hair type, your hair texture, and your own personal look and style is not about following trends, and it's not about a total transformation; it's about working with what you have and making the most of it.

Defining Your Style

Because hair is so tied to self-image, and because it has such power to project that image to others, women obsess about it like few other aspects of their appearance. What's funny is that although our hairstyles can change radically over the years, our attitudes stay pretty much the same. Whether you're high-, low-, or no-maintenance, you'll probably find that your every-day approach to hair fits into one of the following two philosophies.

Understanding which category you fall into helps you better communicate with your stylist so that you can leave the salon happy, not sighing, "Oh, well, it'll grow back."

- ✔ **Free and easy:** You believe that hair should never look like you tried too hard. That doesn't mean that you don't make any effort — because you do — but all the world sees is hair that's never contrived or tricky. It can be short or long, colored or completely natural, but the common denominator is attitude: unflashy, unfussy, and never too far out of line with nature.

  Icons of this type of hairstyle include Katharine Ross, Brigitte Bardot, Grace Kelly, Ava Gardner, and Katharine Hepburn.

- ✔ **Always styled:** You believe that hair *should* look like you tried. After all, flaming red locks, geometrically precise bobs, and perfect chignons don't just happen. Maybe you feel that your natural hair just doesn't express your personality. Maybe having very styled hair makes you feel more pulled-together. For whatever reason, you like lavishing attention on your hair — and calling others' attention to it, too.

  Icons of this type of hairstyle include Ann-Margret, Marilyn Monroe, Veronica Lake, and Elizabeth Taylor.

Keeping It Personal

In addition to figuring out your basic hair philosophy — whether you keep it natural or always have a "style" — you also need to consider some other factors when deciding on a hairstyle:

- ✔ **Your lifestyle:** A busy executive who always needs to look polished will have a clearly different style from a college student who doesn't need to make an impression with her appearance on a regular basis. Think about how you spend the majority of your day, and choose your hairstyle accordingly.

- ✔ **Your personality:** Any hair change needs to be in line with who you are and what your style is — you know whether you like short hair or prefer long hair.

- ✔ **Your age:** Obviously, if you're a young girl, your hair should be in line with your age: simple and natural. As you get older, you can begin playing with hairstyles, colors, and styling techniques. See "Looking Great at Any Age" later in this chapter for more helpful guidelines.

- ✔ **Your mood:** Some days, the urge to do something playful, sexy, or sophisticated with your hair just hits you. You don't necessarily need a whole new haircut — just get creative with your styling products and tools (read Chapter 8 for ideas).

✔ **Your destination:** Pulling your hair into a ponytail is great for the weekend — and not so great for an important board meeting. Like it or not, your hairstyle says a lot about who you are and the impression you're trying to make.

✔ **The weather:** If you've ever tried to straighten curly hair or vice versa, you know all about the weather's effects. Whenever the air is very humid or very dry, your hair may not behave the way you want it to. In this case, don't fight it; go with it.

✔ **The season:** Hair typically gets lighter and freer in summer, while the less-humid days of winter are perfect for trying sleeker styles or for experimenting with deeper tones.

✔ **Time of day:** Although lines between "day hair" and "evening hair" don't really exist these days, doing something different for a night out certainly makes you feel more special. You don't have to do anything elaborate — adding a little fullness or going for a simple updo (see Chapter 8 for how-tos) may be all you need.

✔ **Proportion with your face and body:** If you have a very fine, small face, a head of Big Hair is going to overwhelm you. Larger faces can take more voluminous styles. But imagine a 5-foot-tall woman with a 3-foot fall of hair. Your hairstyle needs to be in balance with your look from head to toe.

✔ **Your styling skills:** Your stylist can give you the most exquisite cut ever, but if you don't have the skills to keep it up, you won't be happy with the way it looks when *you* do it.

Looking Great at Any Age

Your hair changes dramatically throughout your life, but because the process is so slow, you can easily lose sight of the subtle changes that occur over a period of years. This section gives you a helpful hair timeline.

Teens

Hair is usually as healthy as it will ever be during the teen years. This period is also when hairstyling can become an obsession: You undergo your first experiments with cutting, coloring, and styling. Experimentation is understandable, but don't go overboard. As stylist and salon owner Frederic Fekkai puts it, "My advice is to keep your hair as natural as you can, because you know for the rest of your life you're going to mess it up."

✔ Hormonal changes mean that oil production is at its peak during the teen years. If your scalp feels oily, then definitely wash your hair daily, concentrating on the scalp. But resist the urge to overdo: Stripping away all the scalp's oil only pumps up production even more as the sebaceous glands try to compensate.

✔ Beware the bangs-to-face connection. Oils can be transferred back and forth between your hair and your forehead, causing limp, greasy-looking bangs and broken-out skin. Keep your hair off your face as much as possible (use a headband at home, if not at school), and keep both your hair and your skin scrupulously clean. (Chapter 2 tells you how to cleanse your skin; Chapter 5 talks about cleansing hair.)

✔ If you want to play with color, stick to temporary rinses, mousses, or brush-in products. You have plenty of years of highlighting and hair coloring in your future. Right now, just try to enjoy your natural hair color and keep your hair as healthy as possible.

Twenties

Hair goes through many transitions during your twenties because so many changes occur during this period of your life. You get bored with your teenage hairstyle and start playing around. You get out of college and start a career. You may get married and start a family. Keeping a young attitude is great, but you may want to make some subtle changes to make your hair more stylish.

✔ Time and money are key considerations in this decade. Keep it simple: Go for a great cut that keeps its shape between visits, and if you feel the need for color, go low-maintenance. (See Chapter 7 for color options.)

✔ Personal style develops during this decade, and hair is a major part of your look. Although trying new trends is tempting, being true to your own tastes is more helpful. Try to find a style that works for who you are — how you live, how you dress, and how you see your personality.

✔ What really separates the women from the girls: hairstyling skills. Practice until you're proficient at working with your own hair (read Chapter 8 to find out how to get a professional look). Maybe someday you can have a personal stylist on call; until then, you have to know how to do your hair yourself.

✔ Pay attention to changes in the condition of your hair and scalp. As adolescent oiliness subsides, you should probably change to a moisturizing shampoo or add a conditioner to your hair care routine, especially if you're using color or other chemical processes.

Thirties

By now, you have a lot of experience in dealing with your hair, but that doesn't mean you're satisfied. That's because the first signs of age — gray strands, decreasing thickness, flat color — show up during the thirties. If you've resisted coloring your hair until now, suddenly you're running for the Miss Clairol. But you don't need to panic or radically change your look; *small* adjustments in color, cut, and conditioning keep hair looking healthy and beautiful.

- ✔ Color is a great way to perk up hair that's beginning to look dull or flat, but it doesn't have to be a major production. Try a few highlights around your face, or semipermanent color to give your hair more dimension. Both require minimal upkeep, inflict minimal damage, and are a great way to boost volume and shine.

- ✔ With longer styles, taking hair slightly shorter or adding light layers around the face helps counteract the feeling of decreased volume. Removing a bit of the weight lets hair lift from the roots, giving the impression of thicker hair.

- ✔ A common fallacy at this age is that going blonde and growing your hair long makes you look younger. In fact, going blonde may make you look pale or sallow, and long hair can make you look older by dragging your face down. Unless blonde-and-long has been your look all along, it's probably not for you.

Forties

It's not your imagination: Your hair *is* decreasing in thickness, volume, and depth of color — totally natural changes, but not terribly welcome ones. Your hair's growth rate even slows, making length more difficult to attain. Because the difference is so obvious, many women again go to extremes, overprocessing with perms and color to try to restore what's lost. Instead of trying to re-create the hair you had at 25, you're better off to make the most of what you do have while minimizing damage.

- ✔ Instead of perming your hair, get handy with styling aids: thickening and volumizing products to boost body and ease styling; rollers, curling irons, and blow-dyers to enhance lift.

- ✔ Treat your hair with greater care now — especially if you're using any kind of permanent color or process. A gentle shampoo, an intensive conditioner, and occasional deep treatments help restore moisture and shine.

- ✔ If your hair is more than 50 percent gray, you'll probably have to step up to a permanent hair color to get full, lasting coverage. Many women choose to see a pro at this stage, whether for regular visits or to seek advice on at-home color (see Chapter 7 for the whole color story).

- ✔ Red hair is to the forties what blonde hair is to the thirties: the color women reach for as the magic restorer of youth. Again, don't blindly follow the pack. Though red shades are great for warming up a complexion as it grows paler with age, really consider whether that color is *you*. Not sure? A colorist can help you find a great shade.

Fifties

When you hit your fifties, hormones once again play a big role in the appearance of your hair. With menopause, many women experience dramatic, even disturbing, changes: The lack of estrogen can lead to hair fallout. Throughout this decade, hair continues to decrease in thickness and number of strands, and if you've been lucky enough to avoid gray thus far, it's probably on the way.

- ✔ You do not have to cut your hair short once you reach your fifties. If you still have great volume and body, enjoy! But you should keep your hair well-groomed.

- ✔ Going slightly shorter *is* a good idea for two reasons. If your hair has become very fine and thin, having less hair weight maximizes the volume of the hair you have. And if your facial skin is less than taut, long hair can pull it down even further, so shorter is a more flattering option.

- ✔ If you're still coloring your hair with trusty #67, you should probably go a step or two lighter. Your skin's natural pigment continues to fade over time, and too stark a contrast between your skin and your hair looks harsh.

- ✔ As your hair grows progressively more gray — whether it's underneath a color or left *au natural* — your styling skills may need to change. Gray hair can be any texture from wiry to fine, and the texture of your gray hair may be quite different from the texture of your non-gray hair. Style gently, using a volumizing spray to blend the hair types.

- ✔ Hair can feel dry and coarse because the scalp's oil production slows after menopause. Regular conditioning paired with the occasional deep treatment helps restore a supple feel.

Sixties and up

Hair care is just as important now as it ever was. Finer, thinner hair requires its own set of styling rules in order to look its best. And you'd better believe that hair at this age can look _great_ — whether you're still coloring or have finally given into the gray (see Chapter 7 for tips on going gray and keeping it bright).

- ✔ Because skin is at its palest in later years, if you're still coloring your hair, make sure that the color is soft and flattering against your skin tone. Avoid anything unnaturally bright or dark.

- ✔ Gray shows dirt the easiest of all hair colors, so regular, thorough cleansing is a must.

- ✔ Messy, flyaway locks are not attractive on a mature woman, so meticulous grooming is vital — especially if hair is gray. Regular cuts for short hair, or a chic twist for long hair, keep you looking pulled-together.

- ✔ Chlorine, sun, salt, cigarette smoke, perms, and even trace elements in water can give gray hair a yellow cast. To counteract yellowing, care for your hair with specially formulated shampoos and rinses that contain added blue pigment (see Chapter 5).

- ✔ Thinner hair means that the sun can reach the scalp more easily. Be sure to wear a hat or scarf whenever you go to the beach or while walking outdoors in the daytime for extended periods.

Getting Out of a Rut

Looking back on old pictures and realizing that you've had the same exact hairstyle for the past two decades isn't much better than following every new trend. The key is to find a balance. Be aware of what really looks good on you, but also pay attention to what's new. And know that your hair should _always_ be changing as you evolve and change.

You're in a rut if . . .

- ✔ You brag that your last haircut was a year ago.

- ✔ Your favorite drugstore hair color has been discontinued.

- ✔ Your hairstyle hasn't changed since the 1960s.

- ✔ You get your hair done the same way every time you go to the salon because you just don't know what else to do.

- ✔ You consider a ponytail to be "your style."

To get out of a rut . . .

✔ Let a hair-maven friend style your hair.

✔ Go to a salon for a blow-dry or an updo — great for a special occasion.

✔ Part your hair in a different place for one day.

✔ Consider cutting very long hair to the shoulders or letting extremely layered hair grow out to one length.

✔ Try cutting bangs or growing out the fringe that you've had for years.

✔ Go to a wig store and try on a bunch of different looks.

✔ Rip pictures out of magazines that show a cut or color that interests you, and show them to your stylist on your next visit.

✔ Change to a new stylist or colorist.

✔ Buy a different hair color brand or shade.

Finding and Working with a Stylist

Great hair is worth every cent you spend on it, although if you can't afford a lot of cutting and coloring, less is definitely more. That doesn't mean that you have to spend a fortune — everyone knows that "most expensive" does not equal "best" — but one great cut is worth ten mediocre ones.

The first step to finding a new stylist, colorist, or hair technician is to find a salon. There are basically two kinds of salons: *Value salons* emphasize fast, inexpensive haircuts and generally don't require an appointment. They're good for the kids, quick trims, and basic haircuts. *Personal service salons* focus on personal attention and range in prices from reasonable to outrageous. A personal service salon is definitely a better choice for women who want to define their style through haircut and hair color.

Once you decide which type of salon best suits you, you need to find a stylist. The first step is going for a consultation — a five- to ten-minute meeting of the minds. Doing so helps you decide whether this stylist has the same vision you have for your hair, and also helps you figure out exactly what you want and what's really possible. Following is a checklist that you should use not only during your consultation but whenever you go in for more than a simple trim:

✔ **Go in looking like yourself.** Do your hair and makeup as you normally do, and dress in the type of clothes that you most often wear. That way, the stylist sees you the way you appear to the world and gets a good idea of your style.

✔ **Check out the stylist's look.** Is his or her hair a damaged wreck or stuck in a time warp? If a stylist doesn't take good care of his or her *own* hair, you have to wonder how good a job that stylist would do with yours.

✔ **Check out the other clients.** Whether because of word-of-mouth or the area's demographics, most salons end up catering to a certain kind of customer. If you're a trendy 25-year-old, a salon that specializes in roller sets for the over-60 crowd is not likely to give you what you want.

✔ **See whether you feel comfortable.** If the stylist — or the salon — rubs you the wrong way during one short visit, imagine how annoyed you'd be after a couple hours. Pay attention to demeanor — are the people there friendly and really listening to you, or do they seem dismissive? Check out the salon — is the atmosphere pleasant, or does it seem overbooked and disorganized? These are all important indicators of how you'd be treated as a client, so take them seriously. If it doesn't feel right, keep looking.

✔ **Ask whether the stylist is comfortable working with your kind of hair.** You need to work with professionals who are familiar with your hair's unique characteristics. You don't want to find out that someone isn't up to the task after it's too late; be sure to ask up front.

✔ **Know what you want.** The days of sitting down in a chair and saying "Do whatever you like" are over. It's always a good idea to ask the stylist what he or she would do to your hair, but you should have a pretty good idea of what you want. Discuss any ideas, questions, or concerns *before* your hair is wet. Take as much time as you need so that everyone's clear on what you're looking for before you begin.

✔ **Be honest about what you *don't* want.** If your stylist thinks that it's time to cut off all your hair and you're not ready, either just say no or find a compromise somewhere in between if you're curious or interested in making a change.

✔ **Bring pictures.** Says stylist Frederic Fekkai, "I love the idea of a picture, because it opens up the conversation. I'll ask, 'What do you see in this picture? Okay, let's address that with your type of hair, with your shape of face.' It's an education process. It's so important that a woman show you how she wants to look. Even if she comes with a photo that won't work for her, there's something there that captures what she wants — maybe more volume, or a warmer shade — and *that* you can achieve."

Discuss what you like about the photos you bring in. Are you responding to the length or the color? Does the photo show the hair texture you have or the one you *wish* you had? Work together to figure out how to adapt those ideas to your hair, but be realistic — some hair types are just not suited to certain styles.

Don't forget to tip!

For the main stylist or colorist, an average tip is 10 to 15 percent of the fee. For any assistants who helped, a small tip is greatly appreciated. If you're not sure about amounts, ask the front desk for guidance when you're settling up.

✔ **Be honest about upkeep.** Don't commit to a time-intensive 'do if you know that you won't keep it up. If you can't come in monthly to recolor your roots, or if you only want to get a haircut twice a year, say so.

✔ **Let the salon know if you're looking for a color specialist rather than a stylist who does both cutting and coloring.** That way, you can double up on consultation appointments, one for a cut and one for color.

Hair-Cutting Tipsheet

As you think about what hairstyle you want and talk with your stylist about how to achieve that style, you need to focus on two things: the texture and type of hair you have, and the length you want. For example, if you have extremely fine, straight hair, it should probably be cut above the shoulders with some light layering around the face (which gives the illusion of thicker and fuller hair). Following are some other points to consider as you work with your stylist to find a haircut that suits you and your hair type:

✔ **Short hair is not necessarily easier to style.** A short cut that is truly wash-and-wear is rare. There's also more upkeep than with longer hair — you need a trim every four to six weeks to keep short hair in shape.

✔ **Lengths from the chin to just above the shoulder can be flattering on just about every woman, no matter what her age or hair type.** You can customize your cut by keeping it all one length with a blunt edge, cutting layers around the face, or even wearing a stylish bang.

✔ **Bangs soften a high forehead.** Or if you have a long face and want to have hair to your shoulders, a long bang helps balance the length of your hair with the shape of your face.

✔ **Very round or heart-shaped faces look great with long hair.** Whether it's all one length to the shoulder or past the shoulder with some soft layers around the face, this type of haircut is always great for women with straight to wavy, medium, or coarse hair.

- ✔ **Very fine hair should be kept slightly above the shoulder or shorter.** Add layers around the face if necessary to soften.

- ✔ **If you have long hair and are thinking about cutting it considerably shorter, cut off half the amount you and your stylist think should be cut, and then continue to cut.** After you find your length, you can fine-tune it and personalize your style with layers on the sides, long bangs, or rounded edges around the front instead of a straight blunt cut.

- ✔ **Curly hair looks great long if it's full and thick.** Fine or limp curls should be kept shorter, slightly above the shoulder, with light layering around the front to add body.

- ✔ **Be careful not to overlayer the hair.** Layering is best when it's done around the face, not all over the entire head. Many hairstylists think that a lot of layering gives fine, limp hair body or takes the weight out of thick, coarse hair. But in both cases, unless you have a short, tousled haircut, overlayering only looks unkempt and takes away from your hair's natural beauty.

- ✔ **Get regular trims to keep hair ends looking neat.** According to stylist Max Pinell, "If your hair is so fine or damaged that the ends constantly break off, you do need to trim often so the breakage doesn't continue up the hair shaft." How often you revisit the salon depends on how precisely you want to maintain your style; however, says Pinell, "Three months is the longest you should go without a trim."

- ✔ **When you're growing your hair out, trim it as little as possible.** When you go in for a trim, ask your stylist to give you an all-over *dusting,* not a trim or a cut. An all-over dusting takes off only the very ends of your hair to freshen it up.

Trimming your fringe

Because bangs can grow to nuisance length within a few weeks, most salons allow clients to come in for free bang trimmings between appointments. Be sure to call before you drop by to see whether your stylist is at work and able to accommodate you.

If you're pretty handy with the scissors, you can give yourself a slight bang-shaping. The cardinal rule when trimming bangs is *don't do it wet.* You not only obscure how your hair falls naturally, but your hair also shrinks up at least a half-inch after it dries, leaving you with less bangs than you bargained for. Instead, wash and dry your hair as usual, and *then* cut.

To trim your bangs, follow these steps:

1. **Comb your bangs into place, pinning all other hair out of the way.**

2. **Hold your scissors in the proper position for the look you want to achieve.**

   For a blunt, even line, hold the scissors horizontally; for a blurred or layered line, turn them almost-vertical and take small, diagonal snips; for a choppy, imprecise effect, stay vertical and use deeper, angled snips. You can also combine techniques to customize your look even more.

3. **Trim from the center outward *without holding hair down with a comb or fingers*.**

   Pulling or stretching the hair changes the line and makes hair seem longer; after you release the tension, your bangs will be shorter and uneven. If you have a cowlick, take the tiniest possible snips; removing even a little weight from the area can result in a rebound.

4. **Comb your hair back into place often to keep the line together.**

   Go very slowly, recheck often, and remember: Take less rather than more, and don't obsess about a perfectly even line.

Chapter 7
Coloring and Processing Your Hair

· ·

In This Chapter

▶ Finding the hair color, formula, and process that work for you

▶ Working with your colorist to achieve the results you want

▶ Coloring your hair at home

▶ Going back to gray

▶ Perming and straightening your hair

· ·

*H*air coloring has been an obsession for centuries. The Roman "cure" for graying was wearing a paste of earthworms and herbs overnight. Even England's Queen Elizabeth I enhanced her natural red when it began to fade, creating a craze for red hair throughout Renaissance Britain. Modern hair color was born in 1909, when the French Harmless Hair Dye Company (later renamed L'Oreal) successfully invented an easy-to-use formula. Today, estimates show that more than 75 percent of American women color their hair. The question is no longer "Does she or doesn't she?" but "Why not?"

 Not only can hair color cover gray and give you a deeper, lighter, or entirely new shade, when used properly it can add shine, volume, and thickness — actually making your hair look healthier than if it were left untouched. In fact, says hairstylist Max Pinnell, "If your hair's incredibly fine or limp, you *should* color your hair — it actually swells the hair shaft and makes it thicker. A good color job is like having twice as much hair."

Choosing Your Color

Before you put any type of color on your hair, ask yourself this question: Do you want your hair to look very natural — like you don't color it — or do you want hair that's obviously colored? The most important thing to remember when deciding on a hair color is that your hair color is meant to enhance your skin tone and eye color.

For example, if you have dark hair and light eyes and you go blonde, suddenly your eyes lose their drama and your skin looks washed out. Don't forget, Marilyn may have gone platinum blonde, but she started out dirty blond. Nine times out of ten, the closer you stay to your natural shade, the less you'll have to worry about throwing off your skin tone and eye color.

Hair-Coloring Tipsheet

I've created a tipsheet that took me years of trial and error to learn. Some may apply to you and some may not, but the more you know about hair coloring and how it affects your skin, hair, and eyes, the easier it is to find a hair color that's perfect for you.

✓ **The color already in your hair affects any color you put on it.** This goes for whether the color is natural or is left over from a previous color service. (This is why dark hair + blonde hair color = orange. You wind up somewhere in the middle.) Any color you add complicates matters, because you have to deal with the dye left on your hair *and* the chemicals used to put them there. If you color at home, stay with the same types of formulas to avoid incompatibilities; if you go to a pro, be up-front about what's been done to your hair.

✓ **The condition of your hair affects any color you put on it.** The more damaged and porous your hair, the more color it absorbs, resulting in a darker color than you bargained for. This is big problem if only certain areas of the hair are damaged: grown-out ends or highlighted streaks. Color will take there more intensely, leaving you with unwanted lowlights or a line of demarcation.

✓ **Light shades make hair look finer.** The lighter the hair, the finer the texture looks, so if your mane is overly thick, going lighter is a great way to create the illusion of less hair — and to open up your face. If you have fine hair, avoid going too light, because you'll lose definition around your face and hairline and visually decrease your hair's volume.

✓ **Deeper shades make hair look thicker.** More pigment means more presence, which is a great way to boost the appearance of thin hair. However, this technique works only to a point. If your hair is very sparse — meaning very few hairs in total — going too dark creates a marked contrast between your scalp and the air space between hairs.

✓ **Blonde hair does not necessarily look younger.** Women commonly reach for this crutch after "a certain age." But a too-light shade drains more color from your face, leaving you wan and washed-out. In fact, says colorist Bryan Thomson, "As soon as you put a little more depth back into too-blonde hair, it's amazing how it brightens the face — especially the eyes."

✔ **Darker hair does not necessarily look younger.** Because your complexion grows progressively lighter over the years, going darker makes you look *more* pale, not more youthful — even sticking to the color you had when you were younger looks harsh against your paler skin. Going a few shades lighter than your natural color helps keep everything in balance as you age.

✔ **Extreme blonding is almost impossible to maintain.** Heavy-duty bleaching of the hair is unbelievably damaging — and eventually your hair just can't take it anymore. Know going in that you'll have to prepare for the consequences: either a careful growing-out phase with gentler color easing the transition or chopping off the damage altogether.

✔ **Dark dyes are almost impossible to remove.** If you think that you want to go darker, do so *gradually* and use non-permanent products — dark, permanent colors won't budge if you ever want to lighten back up. Your only recourse for too-dark hair is professional, and very damaging, color correction — stripping out the dye with remover or high-powered bleach.

✔ **Hair should never be one solid color.** Because natural hair contains variations of light and dark — even black hair has different tones woven throughout — hair that lacks those variations looks obviously dyed. Home colorists usually inflict this problem on themselves. Trying to make sure that those gray hairs are good and covered, they leave color on too long or use too dark a shade, resulting in a shoe-polish effect. If less time and lighter shades don't help, see a pro to have your color corrected.

✔ **If you get highlights, you don't need to highlight your whole head.** Says colorist Bryan Thomson, "You don't need highlights in the back of your head; you just need them around your face. They're not a substitute for color. If you want to go lighter all over, that's a job for permanent color. The whole concept of highlighting the hair is that it's a low-maintenance, natural-looking enhancement." Done properly, highlights are a great way to brighten your face, add texture and dimension to the hair, and emphasize the lines of your haircut. And if you go just a few shades lighter than the rest of your hair, you only have to redo the highlights about every three months.

✔ **Your shade should change slightly with the seasons.** Because the light in summer and winter is so different, a shade that's gorgeously deep in December can look unnaturally dark in July. Other factors to consider include changes in skin tone (paler in winter, warmer in summer) and even your wardrobe — in winter, for example, darker colors and more clothing around your neck change your hair's whole look. A few well-placed highlights or a slight shift in tone keeps your color in sync with the season.

> ✔ **If you have light hair, be careful when using temporary colors.** Darker shades may not wash out thoroughly — or at all — especially if your hair is porous or damaged.

> ✔ **Take hair color step-by-step.** Unless you have the kind of mindset and lifestyle that are *laissez-faire* about major hair changes, you're better off easing into a new color over a period of months. That way, you can stop when you reach the right point instead of having to backtrack when you've gone too far.

Finding Your Formula

You can change your hair color in basically two ways: by coating the hair shaft with color or by penetrating the hair shaft with bleaching agents and/or dyes. How much and how permanent of a color change you want determines what type of product you or your colorist should use. Table 7-1 breaks down the available products for easy reference — the pros, the cons, and the all-important facts on how much gray you can expect each product to cover, based on the percentage of your hair that's already gray.

Table 7-1		Hair Color Formulas		
Type	*Lasts*	*Gray Coverage*	*Positives*	*Negatives*
Temporary (or rinse)	1 shampoo	Up to 10%	No-commitment way to play with color; good for toning light hair shades, hiding roots between color appointments, or subtle shade enhancement	Can run or rub off; can't lighten hair; may stain very light or porous hair; can discolor the scalp
Semipermanent	Up to 12 shampoos	Up to 20%	Leaves only a slight color deposit on hair; washes out gradually; leaves no roots; good for toning, enhancing color, and using between color services	Can't lighten hair; may leave a stain on lighter shades

Table 7-1 *(continued)*

Type	Lasts	Gray Coverage	Positives	Negatives
Demipermanent (or gloss)	Permanently	Up to 50%	Gently blends away gray; contains less peroxide and dye than permanent formulas; doesn't leave obvious roots; enhances the thickness of fine hair; a great way to refresh or enrich a shade, even out unbalanced color, or tone too-pale or brassy highlights; clear glosses boost hair's shine without depositing color	Little lightening ability; less color intensity than permanent formulas; slightly damaging to the hair shaft
Permanent	Permanently	Up to 100%	Longest-lasting; can change color dramatically; cuticle-roughing effect adds feeling of thickness of fine hair	Chemicals damage the hair shaft; leaves obvious root grow-out

Whether you color your hair at home or have it done at a salon, knowing the differences among the types of color is crucial to getting the results you want. Unfortunately, with home hair color products, manufacturers have no accepted standard for clarifying what type of product you're looking at, so most companies have their own labeling system. Some divide products into Levels 1, 2, and 3; some boxes simply say, "Lasts 6 (or 12 or 24) Shampoos." Read the box carefully to make sure that you're getting the degree of coverage and permanence you desire.

If you're a first-time home colorist, try using a semipermanent color to start with. This way, any mistakes you may make will be short-lived and less damaging.

Picking Your Process

When you've decided on the color and degree of coverage you want, the next step is to choose a process. Simpler hair coloring processes can be done at home, but you may want to leave serious highlighting and lowlighting to a professional. Table 7-2 can help you decide which process is right for you and whether you should attempt it yourself.

Table 7-2	Deciphering Color Processes	
Process	*Definition*	*Do It Yourself?*
Single-process	A color service in which the final look can be achieved by using one formula. Usually refers to permanent color.	Yes. Single-process formulas (including semi- and demi-permanent) are a great choice for home use, as long as you stay within a few shades of your natural color.
Double-process	Any service where achieving the final look takes two steps. The classic example of double-processing is going from very dark hair to blonde; first, you must strip the majority of color from the hair with a bleaching product, and then you apply the final, permanent color (and tone if necessary).	No. This technique is difficult for even pros to do well.
Highlighting	Lightening selected strands of hair as opposed to dyeing the entire head. You can highlight with any color that's lighter than what's already there. Strands are often wrapped in foil to keep them separate during processing (which is why highlighting is also known as *foiling*).	Only if you use a non-bleach product, go just a couple shades lighter, and color just a few strands around your face. Otherwise, go to a pro.
Lowlighting	The opposite of highlighting. Deeper-toned strands are woven throughout the hair to give color more depth and dimension. Often used as a repair technique for overlightened hair.	Not recommended. Darker shades are very difficult to remove, especially from overprocessed strands.

Process	Definition	Do It Yourself?
Toning	The use of temporary, semi-, or demipermanent color to play up or eliminate tones. In salons, toning is the finishing step for hair that's been lightened dramatically. For example, if hair's too brassy after highlighting, a colorist applies an ash-hued toner to dampen the red. The key is using a product that's *less permanent* than the one used to create the color in question.	Sure. Say you used permanent color at home and the results are too ash. Apply a warm-toned color that's less permanent (in this case, demi- or semipermanent or temporary) to help neutralize the drabness. Less-permanent products are also great for toning unwanted shades in natural, non-colored hair.
Filling	The use of color, conditioner, or both together to "fill" porous hair (either in certain areas or all over the head) prior to the application of the final color formula. Helps very damaged, overprocessed hair hold color better and get even, uniform results.	No. If hair is this damaged, a pro should handle all coloring.

Working with Your Colorist

Going to a professional colorist is always a good decision no matter what type of look you're trying to accomplish. However, don't feel that you can surrender all responsibility: Any mistakes are, quite literally, on your head, so you must work in partnership with your colorist to get the results you're looking for. Just as with a haircut, the best way to open up the lines of communication is to *bring pictures*.

"It's very good to bring in pictures from magazines," says colorist Bryan Thomson. "Even if you can't find one that shows exactly what you want, bring in pictures of what you *don't* want because they'll help you establish a common language with your hairdresser. If you show me a picture and say, 'I just hate it when I see this red tone,' and it's a tone I would consider gold, I'll know to stay well away from that because you'll see that as red."

Remember, even though a pro technically can give you any hair color you want, a responsible colorist will not make a drastic change that's going to wreck the condition of your hair. "There are women who go from salon to salon with a picture of a color that is just never going to work for them," says Thomson. "Sometimes you just have to say, 'You know what, you're looking for the impossible, because even if I got it to that color, your hair just wouldn't be able to cope. So let's talk about what you really *can* have, and we'll find something that will be good for you *and* your hair.'"

A few more things to keep in mind before you sit down in the colorist's chair:

- ✔ **Remember that hair color is a time-consuming process.** Allot two to four hours start to finish when you're having your hair color done, especially if you're having highlights. Or if you do a single process and it comes out too dark, you'll need to lighten it, and that's another process and will take even more time.

- ✔ **Be honest about what's been done to your hair.** That includes everything: home color, perms, the works. The longer your hair, the longer those things stick around; even if you did something six months ago, you have to 'fess up. Your colorist *must* know your hair history to prevent disasters, particularly if you've used a henna product or anything containing a metallic dye. As long as the colorist knows what he or she is up against, you should get a good color result.

- ✔ **Find out the salon's policy for fixing a hair color you're unhappy with before you proceed.** The vast majority do not charge for correcting their own color mistakes or hair color you don't like.

- ✔ **Discuss your long-term color plan.** If you're contemplating an entirely new color, tell your colorist so that he or she can plan in advance. Says colorist Bryan Thomson, "If you're a redhead — and I've been keeping your color really bright and saturated — and suddenly you tell me, 'I want to be blonde now,' that's much more work and more potential damage to the hair. Had you told me you wanted to be a blonde by summer, we could have planned and slowly moved you in that direction."

- ✔ **Ask your colorist to recommend a home hair color product.** You may not have the time or money to get your hair professionally colored every six weeks, so you'll need something to keep your color looking good between visits. Your colorist can suggest a product line that's compatible with your needs and with the color products she uses on your hair.

- ✔ **If you travel frequently, ask your colorist for a copy of your formula.** That way, instead of having to home-color in a hotel bathroom during that big business trip, you can go to a salon and have it done. Be warned: Some colorists feel that it's their "intellectual property," but most will give it freely because preventing mistakes makes both your lives easier.

✔ **Make the most of your time in the salon.** Have a manicure. Eat your lunch — some salons have a cafe, and others will send someone to pick up a sandwich for you; or grab something on the way. Make a phone call, catch up on your reading, whatever. Use that time productively and you won't feel like you've wasted part of your day.

Checking Your Color

I've had so many hair color disasters. Now I know exactly what to look for to see whether color's been done well and suits me.

First of all, if you're at a salon, *always* dry your hair before you leave. Don't walk out with wet hair and assume that the color's going to be okay. After you dry it, if you feel like your hair just looks completely colored, like with shoe polish, be honest with yourself — and the colorist — and have it fixed.

If the overall color seems fine, the next thing to do is check to see whether your tips are darker than the roots of your hair. If so, that's a problem. Your ends should be the same shade or even a little lighter than top of the head. That's natural.

Take a mirror and look at the back of your hair. Do you see any spots? Spots can appear if your hair grabs more color in one area than another. If you've had highlights, make sure that they're the color you want them. If they're too light, it's very easy to soften them with an all-over colored gloss.

The last thing to check is the overall tone: Look for very gray or green, ashy tones — especially with blondes — and be very careful about red. Going red is easy if you're a brunette, but it can easily be too brassy, which isn't attractive next to the skin.

If you notice a problem, don't leave without having it taken care of. It's easy to feel intimidated and say to yourself, "It's not that big of a deal" — but it *is* a big deal. Your hair affects how you look and how you feel about yourself. Listen to your instincts. Even if you don't notice a problem the first day, that doesn't mean it's right. Sometimes I have to live with a new hair color or highlight for a day to know whether there's a problem. Either way, you have to tell your colorist that you're not happy and get it fixed immediately.

Coloring Your Hair Yourself

Many women take the do-it-yourself approach to hair color at some point, even if it's just between salon visits. You'll do just fine if you remember one ironclad rule: Don't try to get too sophisticated. Leave major changes to a professional. If you've always done your color yourself and feel comfortable doing it, you're probably using hair color for pretty straightforward reasons: to cover gray, to enhance your natural color, to boost your hair's body, or to save money.

With home hair color, you're better off using the *least permanent* type of product that still gives you satisfactory results. Say you've used semipermanent color for a few years, but now you find that it just doesn't cover your gray as well as you'd like. That's your cue to step up to demipermanent. *Don't* make the big leap into permanent color until it's really necessary. Remember, the less permanent the product, the less chance you have of making a very obvious, lasting mistake.

What you need

Home hair coloring is infinitely easier if you have the right tools — including some useful extras that help speed up the job:

- **Latex or vinyl gloves:** The gloves in hair color kits inevitably tear, and you don't want to go without. Most drugstores or beauty supply stores stock latex or vinyl gloves by the box (around $10 to $20 for 100); look for powder-free, which are less irritating to skin. If you rinse them well, you can reuse the gloves a few times, making them a very economical investment.

- **A color-application brush:** Ideal for touching up roots. You can get a professional version for about a dollar from a beauty supply store (look for a pointed end to aid sectioning), or just get a 3-inch-wide brush with pliable nylon bristles at the hardware store. Make sure that the brush has no metal on it — metal reacts with hair color chemicals — and that no one takes it to paint the garage-door trim.

- **A plastic or glass bowl:** If you're mixing two colors or just want better access for brushing-on purposes, squeezing the goop into a bowl makes things much easier.

- **Plastic hair clips:** For sectioning hair. Again, metal is not recommended.

- **A timing device:** Your watch, a clock, or a kitchen timer.

- **Old towels and an old bathrobe or T-shirt:** Anything that can get dripped on and stained.

- **Optional items:**

  - *Scissors* for snipping the tops off developer bottles

  - A *comb* to make hair-sectioning easier

  - A *hose extension* for the faucet to make rinsing easier

Home hair color tipsheet

- If your goal is to hide gray or heighten your real color, use a product that's one or two steps lighter than your natural shade. You'll avoid the dreaded shoe-polish effect and get nice dimensionality to your color.

- Any type of color stronger than temporary comes with two components: the color itself (usually the smaller vial) and the developer (which activates the color for use on the hair). If you're buying at a beauty supply store, be sure to get both — they're often sold separately — and read labels carefully to be sure that you're pairing the right products. (*Don't* mix brands; that's a recipe for disaster.)

- You *can* mix colors from the exact same product line (in other words, Loving Care with Loving Care or Preference with Preference) to create a more customized shade. It's a great way to individualize color, but don't turn mad scientist: Two shades are plenty. The best approach is to use colors half-and-half in one bottle of developer, saving the remaining color and the second bottle of developer for next time.

- Hair color keeps for six weeks after it's been opened; just don't mix it with developer until you're ready to use it. Once color's mixed, it cannot be stored and may rupture its container, so promptly rinse any extra down the drain.

- If you have long hair, get two boxes of color — or four if you're mixing. You don't want to be caught short and get uneven results.

- Use a clarifying shampoo for a couple days before coloring to remove any product residue or build-up on your hair: It'll help color penetrate better.

- If you have really porous, damaged hair, give yourself a good conditioning treatment *before* you color — you don't want the ends to say "Oh! Something to latch onto!" and wind up darker than your roots. You can also cover your ends or old highlights with conditioner before applying hair color to keep your hair from absorbing too much color.

- Don't color your hair if your scalp is irritated, red, broken, or sore, and don't vigorously brush your hair before coloring: It can irritate and sensitize the scalp.

- Don't worry about matching your eyebrows to your hair: That idea is as old as matching your shoes to your purse. However, if you want to make a change, Chapter 14 has the steps for using brow color.

- If you're unsure about what you're doing before, during, or after, call the manufacturer's toll-free hotline (listed on the instruction sheet or box).

Applying hair color

The first step is always to *read the manufacturer's directions carefully:* Products vary so much that you can never assume that you know the right protocol. When you finish reading, get your gear, get your color mixed and ready to go, and then get down to business:

1. **Smooth a layer of petroleum jelly or thick moisturizer along your hairline.**

   Don't get it into your hair; it prevents color from penetrating. You just want to protect your skin.

2. **Divide the hair into sections and then apply color one section at a time.**

   Start with the most resistant area to give the color more time to work. (With light hair, that's probably the hair at the back and underside of the head; for dark hair, it's usually where there's the most gray.)

   • With a **first-time application**, apply color to the entire length of the hair for the full amount of time. Work section by section from roots to ends to ensure even application.

     If you're having trouble working color all the way to the ends, use your hands to apply a little warm water to the hair; it'll thin the hair color slightly and make it easier to move.

   • With a **touch-up application**, apply color to the roots first and then pull it down the length of the hair for only a few minutes before washing it out. Even if you're using a different or lighter shade than you've used before, *don't put it all over your head until the very end.* The tips always grab more color, and you'll get uneven results. If you're trying to go lighter but the ends aren't cooperating, see a pro.

   "The worst thing at-homers do is run permanent color through the whole head every time they apply," says colorist Bryan Thomson. "It makes the hair much more porous so it grabs more color, and all those layers of color build-up decrease the health of the hair. You're better off to refresh with semipermanent hair color rather than using permanent color over and over."

3. **Immediately wipe excess hair color from your skin to prevent staining. (Don't forget to wipe behind your ears!)**

   Use a cotton pad dampened with water or shampoo, or if your skin's already stained, apply more color over the stained area and quickly wipe it off. (Most beauty supply stores carry special stain-removing products, too.)

4. Check your hair periodically while the color's on.

Remember, the manufacturer's recommended time allotment is a suggestion, not a law. If your hair is damaged or porous, leave color on for less time; if your hair is resistant, coloring may take longer. *Always* do a strand test first so that there are no surprises.

Keep in mind that hair color develops and penetrates faster in the presence of heat. If you're in a steamy bathroom, you may want to cut your time by a few minutes, or if you have very resistant hair, trapping body heat under a plastic shower cap can help speed things along.

5. When time's up, rinse your hair *very* thoroughly.

Rinse until the water runs clear, and then rinse for a few minutes more, wriggling your fingertips gently at scalp level to ensure that every last bit of color is gone.

6. Finish with conditioner.

You don't have to use the one that the manufacturer encloses in the kit (though they usually work well); just be sure that you use something. Your cuticle needs a little TLC after being roughed up by hair color.

7. Jot down what you did as a reminder for next time.

If you tried something new, write down the shade name(s) or number(s) — or snip the infomation from the box panel — and how long you left it in your hair. If you like your results, you'll want a quick reference for when you recolor; if you hate it, you'll want to remember what to avoid (and what to tell a colorist if you need to have it corrected).

If you use a dark hair color shade, throw a towel over your pillow the first night after coloring, or use an old pillowcase that you don't care about. Dark color inevitably transfers until the hair's been washed again, and you don't want to stain your linens.

Maintaining Your Color

No matter whether your new hair color cost $6.99 or $300, you want to invest extra care to keep it looking good. Proper post-color treatment can help your hair color retain its just-done look longer — and even extend the time between color visits. A few important dos and don'ts:

 ✔ **Avoid exposing your hair to sunlight.** The sun's rays have a strong bleaching effect that can wreak havoc with hair color. Though *plenty* of products claim to shield the hair from sun, testing has yet to prove that they protect the hair in the same measurable way that sunscreen protects the skin. Try them if you like, but keep in mind that the only surefire way to safeguard your hair is to wear a scarf or hat, especially at the pool or the beach.

✔ **Avoid exposing hair to chlorinated or salt water.** Everyone knows that blondes can get green hair from too much time in the pool; that's due to copper and other elements present in the water. What you may have overlooked is that chlorine is a potent bleach that can react with *any* hair color in unpredictable and unflattering ways. Saltwater can also ruin hair color; it's harsh and drying, and hair color just can't stand up to the assault. If you're heading out for a swim, slather your hair with conditioner and then cover it with a close-fitting bathing cap.

✔ **Use color-added shampoos and conditioners.** Because they deposit a small amount of dye onto the hair shaft, they help your hair color stay rich and radiant.

✔ **Use products with a slightly acidic pH.** Because hair color uses an alkaline pH to open the hair's cuticle and deposit color, using an acidic pH helps re-close the cuticle, restores the hair's smooth feel, and aids in color retention. An acidic finishing rinse or blast of cold water also helps close the cuticle.

✔ **Avoid clarifying, body-building, and dandruff shampoos.** These products can strip the hair — especially if it just went through a major hair color process — and contain little or no conditioning ingredients. If flakes are a problem, use a dandruff shampoo only as often as really needed — perhaps once a week.

Going with the Gray

There comes a point in the hair color battle when it's clear that the gray has won, so rather than color, color, color for decades, many women finally let their hair go gray. Gray hair does not automatically enroll you in the Old Lady Club. On the contrary, gray is incredibly chic when kept bright, beautiful, and well-groomed.

Hair goes through many stages as gray grows in. The word *gray* is, in fact, a misnomer: Because these strands lack pigment, they're actually white; what creates the spectrum of gray shades is simply the proportion of colorless to colored hair. White strands first become really noticeable at the salt-and-pepper stage, when hair's gray-to-pigment ratio is about 50/50. Most pros agree that hair must be at least 50 percent gray, and the remaining color relatively dark, for a salt-and-pepper look to work. Over time, the pigmentless strands overtake the pigmented strands, and the hair progresses through shades of slate and silver on its way to pure white.

So how *do* you go gray after years of using permanent color? Start by checking out the how-tos in this section.

Changing from colored hair to gray

If your gray is not terribly noticeable (say, less than 30 percent, or blended with very light hair), you *can* stop coloring altogether as long as your roots aren't obvious. However, those cases are rare, so here are a few ways to make the switch:

- ✔ Touch up your hairline and roots with a temporary or semipermanent color as you let the permanently colored hair grow out. After several months and several trims, all the old color will be gone — and when you stop using the temporary formula, your hair reverts to its uncolored state.

- ✔ If you have very dark hair, go lighter and less intense with your hair color shade over a period of months, and then go the route just outlined. Your colorist can help the process along by adding highlights that help lift your color even more.

- ✔ If you have light hair, have your colorist place an ever-decreasing number of highlights in your hair. As they grow out, your gray grows out with them, and eventually highlighting can cease altogether.

- ✔ If you're certain that you're almost completely white under your hair color, a skilled colorist can remove the added pigment and save you a lot of growing-out grief. However, this process is quite rough on the hair and may not remove dark dyes completely, so discuss the pros and cons thoroughly first.

After your gray is out in the open, you need to make a few simple changes to help it look its best. The whiter your shade, the more important upkeep becomes. It's kind of like hair's version of a new white T-shirt: Treat it with care and you'll help it retain its fresh look.

Gray hair tipsheet

- ✔ As more gray strands grow in, you may notice that they have a different texture than your pigmented hair. Also, as you age, your hair becomes thinner and more sparse. Both things can take some getting used to — sometimes it's like having all-new hair — so you need to brush up on your styling skills. (Your stylist can help with suggestions.)

- ✔ Very white hair can make the skin appear drained of color, so alter your makeup application accordingly. (Be sure to read Part III, which tells you everything you need to know about makeup.)

- ✔ Gray hair must be kept absolutely clean because it shows dirt and oil more quickly than any other shade, especially near the roots.

✔ A yellowish cast to the hair is a classic sign that impurities have been absorbed — usually from smoke, pollution, chlorine, or water-borne particles. Stepped-up cleansing can help to a point, but to really neutralize the yellow tone, you need to use a shampoo, conditioner, or rinse that contains either blue or violet pigment. (One "blue" product is plenty.)

✔ Avoid excessive heat from blow-dryers, curling irons, and straightening combs. All these styling tools can scorch the hair, leaving visible yellow or brown areas.

✔ Steer clear of hair care or styling products that have a bright or deep color. The dyes that give a product a signature shade — a bright pink hair gel, for example — can leave a stain on white hair that can be difficult to remove.

✔ Gray hair *must* be kept under control. Shoulder length or shorter is usually best.

✔ Just because you've gone gray doesn't mean that hair color can do nothing for you. If you feel that your hair looks too mousy, too ashy, or too dull, see a colorist. A colorist can add highlights or lowlights to give your hair more depth, tone your gray to a more flattering shade, or enhance your hair's shine with color-free gloss. (Color-tinkering really is best left to the pros — mistakes on gray hair can be obvious.)

Perming and Straightening

The only truly effective way to permanently change your hair's natural curl (or lack thereof) is to break the bonds that create your hair's shape with highly alkaline chemicals, reshape it into the desired configuration, and then re-form the bonds with a neutralizing solution so that your hair hardens into the new shape. All chemical formulas used for perming and straightening work this way, and if you think that their action sounds harsh, you're right.

Though formulations have come a long way over the last generation, these products are still extremely hard on the hair and absolutely *not appropriate* for at-home use — no matter how adept you think you are or how much money you want to save. These processes involve a highly complicated set of variables, from judging your hair's health and degree of resistance to choosing the best product, applying it evenly, and timing it right. It's tricky even for professionals to pull off, so finding a skilled technician is imperative if you're considering either of these services.

✔ **Perm or straighten *before* using hair color,** because the strong chemical formulas have a color-fading effect. The recommended waiting time between processes is at least 48 hours — and permanent hair color, bleaching, metallic dyes, and henna-based products are *not* recommended for chemically processed hair. Most pros prefer semi-permanent hair color in this situation. Because it is applied over a roughed-up cuticle, it usually has more staying power.

✔ **Deep-condition porous or damaged hair before processing.** A compromised cuticle absorbs more of anything that's put on it, chemicals included, and that can create uneven or unsightly results. Check out Chapter 5 for deep-conditioning tips and how-tos.

✔ **Have a couple of pre-service clarifying shampoos.** Residue from sticky or greasy styling products and hard water can prevent chemicals from penetrating evenly. Using an anti-residue shampoo removes unwelcome build-up and ensures more-uniform processing.

✔ **Cut hair *after* chemical processing** so that the style is designed for the hair's new shape. However, if you're planning to go radically shorter, your stylist should cut your hair to approximately the right length and then do the final cutting after the processing is complete.

✔ **Processing chemicals can burn the scalp, skin, and eyes.** If your scalp is sensitive or broken in any way, do not use chemicals. Don't vigorously brush your hair before a chemical service, either — doing so irritates the scalp. If you feel a burning sensation on your scalp or skin, rinse out the formula *immediately*. And if any chemicals get into your eyes, flush immediately and thoroughly with water and see a physician right away.

✔ **Know how long chemicals should be left on your hair.** In a busy salon, your pro may not hear your timer go off — and sitting there in overtime with a head full of chemicals is a *very* bad idea. Keep track of time yourself, and alert your technician when time's up.

✔ **Redoing an unsuccessful service *is* possible, but it's not easy to do well, and it's certainly not easy on your hair.** If you didn't get the degree of curl or straightness you wanted, discuss your options with your technician — and realize that you're opening yourself up to a lot of potential damage.

✔ **Treat hair with great care after chemical processing.** Provide your hair with gentler shampoo, stepped-up conditioning, and protection from heat, mechanical styling, sun, and chlorine. The tips in "Maintaining Your Color" earlier in this chapter are equally appropriate for chemically processed hair, so flip back and take a look.

Still want better hair through chemistry? Read on — I discuss the methods and merits of each process so that you can make a truly informed decision.

Perm particulars

No one "needs" a perm, nor is curly hair in any way better, prettier, or more feminine than straight hair. Maybe curls are more "you" and you've had it with rollers. For you, a perm *is* easier on a day-to-day basis, but know that you're harming your hair every time you get one. However, if you're simply looking for body, perms should be a last resort. With today's advanced haircutting techniques, styling appliances, and products, subjecting your hair to all that damage isn't necessary.

Salon owner and stylist Frederic Fekkai doesn't believe in perms. What he will do for very flat hair that's hard to work with is a root perm on the top of the head, the hairline, and the crown. It gives great body and volume, but you never see a perm.

Perm formulas

Perms use two chemical formulas to do their work: a waving solution to break the hair's bonds and a neutralizing solution to set the newly curled shape. (Some neutralizers even include semipermanent color.) Following are the most-used waving formulas; the one your technician uses will depend on the health of your hair and the look you want to achieve.

- **Alkaline perms** use a strongly alkaline chemical ingredient (ammonium thioglycolate) and tend to give the fastest and longest-lasting results. They're best for hard-to-curl hair or for creating a strong or tightly curled effect.

- **Acid-balanced perms** utilize a gentler chemical (glyceryl monothioglycate) and a lower pH. Though not as harsh as alkaline perms, they must be left on longer and activated with heat. *Endothermic* formulas need a heat source, such as a bonnet-type hair-dryer, to do their work; *exothermic* formulas chemically generate their own heat. Either type is good for fragile or previously processed hair or for softer curl effects.

Perming techniques

Several techniques are used to perm hair. The look you want determines the technique to be used.

- **Traditional perm:** Curling or waving the entire head of hair. Though rods are usually placed horizontally, dozens of configurations are possible, depending on rod size, number, and desired effect.

- **Body wave:** A variation on the traditional perm, with large-diameter rods that create a gentle wave pattern in the hair.

✔ **Reverse perm:** Actually a method of straightening hair, reverse perming uses large-diameter rods to reset tightly curled hair into a looser, more manageable curl pattern.

✔ **Root perm:** Rods are placed at the roots only to give lift and volume or to curl new grow-out when the rest of hair has been permed previously.

✔ **Spiral perm:** Hair is rolled vertically rather than horizontally to create long, corkscrew-type curls.

✔ **Spot perm (or weave perm):** Perm rods are used only in certain areas of the hair to add body where needed.

If you have any qualms about your hair's ability to withstand perm chemicals — especially if your hair has had any kind of previous chemical processing — request that a test curl be done on a lock or two before your whole head is doused in waving solution. After you give the go-ahead, your stylist should check curls regularly, partially unwinding one rod at approximately ten-minute intervals to gauge progress.

Perming tipsheet

✔ Rods make all the difference in a perm's look. They must be rolled into the hair with *slight* tension and should never pull at the roots or hang loosely from the scalp. Hair that's rolled too tightly breaks; hair that's too loose doesn't get a defined, neat curl. Alert your technician to either situation.

✔ Remember, the *size* of the rod determines the size of the curl. Skinny rods create a tight curl, and fat rods create loose curls. The rod's *shape* also affects the final result, because concave rods curl hair tighter at the ends and looser toward the scalp, and straight rods curl uniformly from root to tip. If you see teeny rods and you asked for loose curls, speak up.

✔ Hair can be rolled to redirect growth patterns — a great solution for sweeping hair away from the face or taming a cowlick.

✔ Don't shampoo, condition, or vigorously style newly permed hair for at least 48 hours to give your curls time to set.

✔ If your perm is done well, you shouldn't have to redo for several months. The longer between perms, the better for your hair, but don't let it go too far. Three to four months between perms is average.

✔ The easiest way to grow out a perm is to cut off as much processed hair as possible and then blow-dry hair smooth during the transition period, while getting regular trims.

Straight talk

Chemical straightening (also known as *relaxing*) can make life easier for women with kinky or very curly hair. Though the majority of women who straighten their hair are of African ancestry, chemical straighteners are for anyone with extremely curly or kinky hair. "For some women, no matter what their ethnic background, curly hair just isn't appealing," says salon owner and stylist Frederic Fekkai. "It can get frizzy or out-of-control, and they can't deal with it. Straightening softens up the hair and makes it flatter, so it's much easier to style."

Other benefits to straightening: You reduce or eliminate the need for damaging heat-styling, and you're free to shampoo more frequently because "starting from scratch" with a wet head isn't such a pain in the neck.

Straightening is tempting, but of course there's a catch: You're still going to inflict damage. Straighteners work by breaking down and flattening the hair's cuticle layer, so hair will be drier and more porous afterward and in need of intensive TLC. It's not a decision to be made lightly. Chemically straightening wavy hair to save five minutes a day with the blow-dryer may be overly drastic.

Allow only a *very* experienced professional to straighten your hair. The process is far too involved for the average person to deal with, and misuse of straightening chemicals can leave you damaged at best, bald at worst. Do yourself a favor and forgo the home relaxer kit. Having this process done right is worth every penny.

Straightener formulas

You must know one critical thing about straightener formulas: They absolutely *do not* mix. Follow a sodium hydroxide-based straightener with a thio-type relaxer, and your hair literally turns to jelly and slides down the drain. If you're planning to move or switch salons, ask — and write down — what formula your technician has been using to avoid any chance of a mix-up.

- **Sodium hydroxide**, also known as lye, is the strongest hair-straightening chemical in common use. It efficiently breaks down the cuticle to remove the most curl in the shortest amount of time, and it also gives the longest-lasting effect. Some formulas require a protective "base" during processing: a petroleum cream that shields the scalp and skin from the chemical's caustic effect. Best for resistant or very kinky hair and for creating super-straight looks.

- **Calcium hydroxide** is commonly known as a "no lye" relaxer, but that itself is a lie — it's just a slightly different type. No-lye formulas can leave hair dull and frizzy instead of smooth because their milder action isn't strong enough to break down the cuticle evenly. Not recommended. Most pros prefer sodium hydroxide.

✔ **Ammonium thioglycolate**, or "thio-type" relaxers, use the same active chemical as alkaline perms, but in a heavier cream base. With a lower pH than sodium hydroxide, thio also has a milder relaxing action, so it's often preferred for less-curly hair, less-intensive straightening, or for correcting frizzy perms. Best for moderately curly or fine hair, to soften or gently relax curl, or when you don't want completely straight hair.

Avoid chemical straighteners if your hair has been bleached, permanently colored, or exposed to metallic dyes — the combination can destroy the hair. Straightening is also not recommended if your hair's very damaged or porous. If you're a borderline case, your technician can pretreat your hair with a rich conditioner to smooth over damaged areas and get more even results. In all cases, a strand test must be done.

Straightening techniques

The thing to remember about relaxing the hair is that perfectly straight is not your only option. Before you commit to a technique, discuss your expectations with your technician. If you like having a bit of curve or curl to your hair, going stick-straight and then having to use hot rollers is ridiculous (and damaging). Go for a softer, more relaxed technique instead.

✔ **Straightening:** A strong chemical formula (usually sodium hydroxide) is applied to hair, which then is combed as straight as possible, rinsed, and neutralized to set the shape.

✔ **Relaxing:** This term is often used interchangeably with straightening, but there's a difference. Relaxing the hair can achieve a range of results, from gently smoothing out curl to reducing frizz, in addition to creating straight styles.

✔ **Texturizing (also known as chemical blow-out):** Relaxer is combed through the hair and left in briefly to loosen the curl pattern. The hair is straightened slightly, which makes it look longer and improves manageability.

✔ **Soft curl perm:** This two-part styling method uses thio-type relaxer to reshape the hair's natural curl. First, relaxer is applied and the hair is combed straight until it's softened and flexible. Next, the hair is rinsed and rolled onto perm rods to create a new curl pattern. Thio is reapplied, and then the hair is rinsed again and neutralized to harden into its new form.

When your roots become noticeable (usually in two to three months), it's time for a root retouch. Your technician applies relaxer to the new growth *only* (protecting your previously treated hair with a base or heavy conditioner) to smooth root-area hair. *Don't* try to do this yourself; this process should be left to a pro. If chemicals accidentally overlap onto hair that's already straightened, severe breakage can result.

Straightening tipsheet

✔ Treat straightened hair extra gently. Avoid vigorous brushing and sponge or Velcro rollers that can catch and snap fragile strands, and keep heat-styling to an absolute minimum. Regular deep-conditioning treatments are practically mandatory (see Chapter 5 for types and application tips).

✔ Once you straighten your hair, you must keep it straightened. Not only do curly roots look strange, but the dueling textures make comb-through almost impossible. If you can't get in right away for a root retouch, you can bridge the texture gap by blow-drying or wet-setting to de-kink the roots. Or if you're very dexterous, gently straighten *the roots only* with a flat iron or pressing iron (see Chapter 8 for more on these tools).

✔ Eventually, most women want to give their hair a break from straightening. Speak with your stylist or professional about your options.

Chapter 8

Styling Your Hair

● ●

● ●

*I*n all my years of modeling, whenever I've had to choose between having my hair done or my makeup done, I've always chosen my hair. I've always felt that I could do my makeup but could never really do my hair like a professional stylist.

Over the years, and through watching so many great hairstylists style my hair, I've learned that I can achieve the results I want from my hair at home with a few simple tips and tricks. The key to styling your hair yourself is having the right products and tools. Once you have good products and tools, it's a matter of practicing the right techniques. In this chapter, I define the best tools and products available. You also get tips on styling your hair at home from one of my favorite hairstylists, Max Pinnell.

Assembling Your Toolkit

Using the right hairstyling tools has a tremendous impact on your hair's finished look. The difference between good-enough hair and great-looking hair can be as simple as changing hairbrushes, so it really does pay to know which tools do what, and which work best for your hair. You won't need everything listed in this section, but having a selection of brushes, tools, and styling products on hand is a great way to vary your hairstyle and be prepared for those special occasions.

Styling tools

Having the right styling tools, from brushes to heated appliances, is essential. Your brushes and combs must be the right shape and size to get the job done right. And your heated appliances need to be of good enough quality so that they not only make your job as stylist easier but also last a long time. All these tools are available at beauty supply stores, larger drugstores, and salons. They range in price from very inexpensive to very expensive. This section describes all the available tools, what their functions are, and how to select them according to your hair type.

Brushes

Brushes really serve two functions: grooming and styling. *Grooming* is nothing more than a good brush-through. *Styling,* on the other hand, is all about shaping the hair. Paired with a blow-dryer, the brush is one of the most effective tools in all of hairstyling.

Bristles are a key element to consider. They come in many different materials and degrees of firmness, and it's important to choose those that treat your hair gently yet still offer good control. In general, bristles should be firm enough to penetrate and grip the hair effectively without breaking it — thick hair demands a stiffer bristle than thin hair.

- **Natural bristles**, or boar bristles, are the most expensive. They come in varying degrees of firmness, and although they're considered gentler on the hair than other bristle types, some are stiff and sharp, so check them carefully before you buy. Natural bristles have a smoothing effect on the hair and help distribute oil evenly along the hair shaft — both great for enhancing hair's shine. Boar bristles are also less inclined to produce static than nylon bristles, and are favored by most pros for large-diameter round brushes.

- **Nylon bristles** come in a couple of varieties. The whisker-thin types that mimic boar bristles can be used singly or in tufts, depending on their thickness and firmness, and are often combined with natural bristles to improve brushability. The thicker, stiffer, longer bristle type is typically seen in vent brushes. With either type of bristles, look for rounded or ball-tipped ends so that you don't scratch your scalp.

Perhaps even more important to consider is a brush's size and shape. *Size* matters because the brush must be in line with the hair's length: A tiny brush is great for very short hair but would get lost in thick tresses. Brush *shape* is critical because with certain styling techniques — especially when blow-drying — the shape of the brush creates the shape of the hair. Finding a brush that fits on both counts makes styling easier and more efficient. Here are the most-used types and what they can and cannot do:

✔ **Flat brushes** are the classic oval or rectangle brushes with bristles on one side only. The best have either natural or mixed natural/nylon bristles that are set into a rubber-cushioned base at a slightly curved angle. They're good all-around tools for basic hair-brushing and styling, but not precise enough to curl or straighten hair while blow-drying.

✔ **Vent brushes** have widely spaced bristles and slots or openings on the back of the brush that enable air to flow through. Although this type of brush adds volume to the hair and cuts drying time, it prevents heat from being trapped as effectively as with other brushes, so it isn't great for smoothing frizzy or curly hair.

✔ **Round brushes** have bristles all around the base and come in dozens of sizes; the diameter you choose depends on the length of your hair and what you want to accomplish. Small-diameter brushes can curl, volumize, or straighten short hair. Large-diameter brushes are too big to effectively curl hair — but they can't be beat for straightening it. (For optimum "grab," look for tufts of natural bristles.) A general rule: The brush should be big enough that your hair can't wrap around it more than twice.

✔ **Paddle brushes** are broad and flat with a wide base. Because they have such a large surface area and no curvature, they're great for brushing very long hair quickly and without the threat of it "catching" along the way. They're also helpful for blow-drying long hair that's straight or wavy, but the flat base can't create the pull needed to straighten curly hair. (They're great for finishing hair to a bone-straight look after you blow out curl with a round brush, however.) Look for single, nylon bristles and a rubber cushion at the base to help hair flow through smoothly.

If you're having a hard time finding good brushes in your area, use your stylist as a resource. She'll know which types of brushes work best for your hair and can steer you in the right direction, whether it be a nearby beauty supply store or a telephone order line. (See Appendix B for brush resources as well.)

Combs

Combs come in a variety of sizes and materials. When you're shopping for combs, keep in mind that hard rubber or plastic is usually best. And as a rule, if it hurts your hand, it will probably hurt your scalp. Combs can be used for styling very short hair, but women with locks that are more than a few inches long are usually better off using a brush for styling and a comb for detangling and sectioning. Here are the different types available:

✔ **All-purpose:** Your comb-of-all-trades. Usually found with thinner, close-spaced teeth on one half and thicker, wider-spaced teeth on the other.

✔ **Tail:** Also known as "rattail" combs, so named for their long, pointed end. With their fine, closely spaced teeth, tail combs are ideal for backcombing; the "tail" is used for sectioning and arranging hair into place, especially for curly styles.

- **Teasing:** These combs have alternating long and short, serrated teeth — an effective configuration for pushing hair onto itself in backcombing. Choose a teasing comb according to your hair's thickness; the finer your hair, the closer together the teeth should be.

- **Wide-tooth:** Good for detangling wet hair and dry hair that's very thick or curly. Not really appropriate for styling.

- **Detangling:** Similar in shape to the basic wide-tooth version, but with two S-shaped rows of teeth instead of one straight row for more effective tangle removal.

- **Pick:** Cousins to the comb, picks have long, widely spaced teeth. They're used to give lift and volume to curly or kinky hair. They can also be used to detangle wet hair.

Blow-dryers

Blow-dryers are the key to most hairstyles. Whether you're straightening curly hair or giving body and bend to straight hair, a blow-dryer is essential. Here are some features to consider when buying or using these appliances:

- **1,500 watts minimum:** According to salon owner and stylist Frederic Fekkai, "If your blow-dryer isn't at least 1,500 watts, you'll spend too much time drying your hair — and that's when you end up hurting your hair." But don't go too much higher unless you need it: Very fast, hot air can overwhelm fine or curly hair.

- **Heat and speed settings:** Although not essential, different heat and speed settings are handy for precision styling and straightening.

- **Cool shot button:** This great "extra" is quickly becoming standard on new blow-dryer models: a trigger that instantly turns off the heating element so that the unit blows cool air. It's used as a finishing step, particularly when hair's been styled by using high heat, because cooling the hair helps set its new shape in place — and also closes the cuticle to boost shine.

- **Attachments:** With some styles, attachments are extremely useful for getting great results. Some blow-dryers come with their own; others can be purchased separately and adjusted to almost any size nozzle. Maybe you need them, maybe you don't, but here are a few favorites:

  - **Diffuser:** Disperses airflow so that curls aren't straightened by the air's force. You can find a big selection of diffuser shapes and sizes to choose from — good for slowly drying curly or wavy hair.

  - **Air director:** Found on almost every blow-dryer, this little end-cap narrows at the edges, forcing air to come out faster and in a smaller space. Great for smoothing and straightening the hair.

- **Volumizer:** Relatively new on the scene, these finger-like implements direct air right to hair's roots for extra fluff.

- **Cap:** You attach this nylon bonnet to your blow-dryer nozzle. All caps are made primarily for drying hair in roller sets, but they're also great for warming the hair during deep-conditioning treatments.

Curling and straightening irons

As the saying goes, you always want what you don't have. That's where curling and straightening irons come into play: Both tools help you get the opposite of what's on your head when you're hair's in its natural state.

- **Curling iron:** The classic curl creator. The business end, called the _rod,_ comes in a variety of diameters: Small is good for short hair or making tight curls; large is better for creating looser curls in longer hair, and can even help straighten curly hair in much the same way as a big, round brush. The best curling irons come with variable heat settings, which are a big plus if your hair's either delicate or resistant: You can turn it as low or as high as you need it. Most consumer models come with a spring closure "shell" — the clamp-like piece that holds hair in place during curling — which is definitely a feature that you don't want to be without. Operating a non-sprung handle is much too difficult for a non-pro.

- **Curling brush:** This offshoot of the curling iron has all its predecessor's attributes, plus spiky bristles all the way around the rod. Because the bristles hold hair in place, there's no shell closure to open and shut — an attribute that some women find speeds up the curling process.

- **Straightening irons:** There are two types of straightening irons. Both work the same way, using a combination of heat and tension to iron the curl out of hair. (Use them on dry hair only.) This process is, of course, very damaging, especially if done on a daily basis. Therefore, the best use of these appliances is for finishing the hair after pre-straightening with a blow-dryer.

  - **Flat iron:** This device has two flat, heated plates that open and shut like an alligator's jaws. You clamp hair between the plates and slowly draw the iron down to the ends of the hair. Some models employ mist, but moisture is exactly what you _don't_ want near straightened hair — steam can easily burn the scalp and skin.

  - **Pressing comb:** Also called a _hot comb,_ this device is familiar to women with kinky hair. It resembles a tail comb in shape, is usually made of brass or steel, and can be found with long, widely spaced teeth for long or thick hair or shorter, closely spaced teeth for shorter or finer hair. For home use, electric pressing combs with variable heat settings are best: You can select the lowest temperature that's still effective for your hair.

TIP

Caring for your brushes and combs

Although a well-made brush or comb *will* last a long time, it won't last forever — especially if it isn't properly maintained. And if you use lots of styling products, have very oily hair, or use your tools every single day, you need to clean your tools more often. Here's how:

1. Use a comb to remove all the hair you can from your brushes; this also helps loosen accumulated product residue and scalp flakes from the bristles and base.

2. Fill your sink with hot water and about ¼ cup of shampoo. Add a little white vinegar if build-up is particularly bad.

3. Toss in plastic-handled brushes and hard-rubber combs and leave them to soak for at least ten minutes. Do not soak wooden brushes or brushes with a rubber-cushion base; with these, give the heads a good, quick swish in the water and remove.

4. Rinse well under a running tap, shake out any excess water, and leave out on a towel to air-dry.

Rollers

Not so long ago, rollers (or "curlers") were the only styling option that most women had. If you wanted any kind of hairstyle, you dutifully washed your hair each night before bed, set it all in rollers, and then slept on it overnight. Because there wasn't much of a selection back then, women did some resourceful recycling of rags, orange juice cans, pipe cleaners, and other household items to get different looks. When blow-dryers and curling irons came on the scene, rollers were cast aside as old-fashioned and time-consuming — which, in fact, they were.

Now, things have changed. Rollers are enjoying a kind of renaissance because they're being used as a quick way to enhance a style — not as the only means to create one. Best of all, they're very affordable and come in a wide variety of shapes and sizes.

- **Hot rollers:** Rollers that rest in a base unit that you plug into an electrical outlet. The best ones come with a nonstick or spongy coating that's gentler on hair. These are for use on dry hair only and can be used to create strong curl or a looser curl when used at cooler temperatures. If you find that you created too strong a curl, use a blow-dryer to pull out some of the curl and finish by smoothing a small amount of hair cream all over the hair.

- **Steam rollers:** Sponge rollers that are placed on top of a contraption that emits steam, which heats the rollers. They are the gentlest on the hair and give a beautiful, soft-looking curl. You can use them without steam for just a bend.

✔ **Velcro rollers:** Non-heated rollers that are usually wound into just-damp or dry hair to add a bit of volume. Velcro rollers are a favorite with hairstylists to provide quick lift at the roots. (Velcro rollers are supposedly self-holding, but even the pros hold them in place with roller pins or clips.)

Styling products

Styling products make all the difference in shaping your hair into a new style and creating the texture you want. They can also improve the health of your hair and give your hair unbelievable shine. In choosing the ones you need, keep in mind that *how* and *when* you use a product is just as important as the product itself.

✔ **Anti-frizz serums** work by coating the hair shaft with a very thin layer of silicone, which smoothes and seals the cuticle so that water can't penetrate it — thereby preventing frizz. However, too much product can weigh down the hair, attract dirt, and leave a coating that's difficult to remove, so use these products sparingly. Apply them to wet hair before styling or use them on dry hair to smooth down frizz or flyaways. Hold sprays 4 to 5 inches from hair and apply a light, even mist; with liquids or serums, place a small drop in your palm, rub your hands together, and then run your hands through your hair, starting at the ends.

✔ **Hairspray** coats the hair with a fine layer of resins and other holding agents to keep hair in place and seal out style-wrecking humidity. It's available in many degrees of hold, from very light to super-strong. Hairspray comes in two common forms: aerosols, which go on as a light, quick-drying mist; and pump sprays, which tend to go on wetter and heavier, take longer to dry, and therefore are better for spot application. Use either type sparingly on dry hair, only where needed, after styling. If you're using hairspray, it should be the final styling product that you apply to your hair.

✔ **Gel** comes in a range of different consistencies; generally, the thicker the gel, the more control it gives. Thin, spray-on formulas gently enhance hair's texture and manageability. When used on wet hair, gels are great for creating slicked-back looks, controlling curl, and molding hair into new shapes. On dry hair, gels can be used to accentuate certain areas.

✔ **Mousse:** This lighter-than-air foam adds volume and fullness to fine hair, especially when applied near the roots before blow-drying. It can also be used on dry hair for gentle shaping and control, but use it sparingly or it will flatten the hair.

✔ **Shine enhancers:** Like anti-frizz serums, these products coat the hair shaft with a layer of silicone, which creates a wonderfully glossy finish. (Be sure to apply them with a light touch so that you don't weigh down your hair.) Shine enhancers should be applied to dry hair.

✔ **Styling creams:** High in emollients, these products are similar to leave-in conditioners but have the added styling control of polymers and resins. Applied to wet hair, they're great for helping control curl and smooth frizziness; used on dry hair, they can tame flyaways and help protect hair ends when rollers and other styling implements are used.

✔ **Thickeners and volumizers:** The main ingredients in most of these products are *humectants,* which work to swell the hair shaft, and *polymers,* which coat and separate hairs to create the look and feel of more volume. They're most effective when used near the roots before blow-drying to help create lift in the hair, but they can be applied sparingly throughout very fine hair to help improve texture.

✔ **Curl revitalizers and activators:** These water-and-humectant mixtures use moisture to perk up deflated curls; however, they cannot *create* curl in hair that's not already inclined to do so. For best results, use these products on damp hair.

Helpers and accessories

Styling your hair is much easier if you employ a few of these little helpers along the way. They're great for holding stray locks while you blow-dry, anchoring a roller securely in place, and creating an updo with the greatest of ease.

✔ **Bobby pins** have one straight side and one crimped side and are designed to hold small amounts of hair snugly. For updos, choose a color that's close to that of your hair, and make sure that the pins have rounded, plastic-tipped ends.

✔ **Roller pins** are bigger, stronger, and thicker than bobby pins, and they're used to hold rollers in place. Roller pins are also useful for pinning up larger hair sections while styling, but they're too obvious for use in an updo.

✔ **Hairpins** are thinner than bobby pins, crimped on both sides, and come in a selection of hair-toned colors. Their open U shape can hold larger amounts of hair than a bobby pin, but not as tightly.

✔ **Clips and clamps** are usually found in silvery aluminum or steel and range from single-prong to double-prong, flat to curved. Clips are the smaller of the duo, used to secure small sections in place while drying hair into curled, waved, or straight shapes. (To avoid leaving a dent in the hair, use flat clips.) Clamps are useful for holding rollers in place or sectioning hair during blow-drying. Sizes and shapes vary from slim duckbill clamps (hinged at one end) to larger center-hinged clamps that can hold sizable portions of hair up and out of the way.

✔ **Ponytail holders:** Available in a huge variety of sizes and colors, these must-haves keep hair pulled securely away from the face. The best are thick, smooth circles of elastic with a tightly woven stretch covering; choose a color close to your hair's for the most polished look. A pro favorite: Elastiques elastic bands, a length of covered elastic with hooks on each end that can be custom-adjusted to hair (see Appendix B for information).

✔ **Barrettes:** Made from metal, plastic, or a combination of the two, barrettes come in unlimited colors, shapes, and sizes — from teeny baby barrettes to ones big enough to hold an entire head of hair. If your hair's in fragile condition, beware of barrettes with teeth or sharp, metallic edges at the clasp.

✔ **Hair combs:** Great for creating pulled-back sections or updos, hair combs come in several sizes and colors. The small, thin varieties can be used much like hairpins to hold an updo in place; larger ornamental combs are best for accenting a certain hair section (pulled-back sides, for example) or a finished updo. In any size, the best have smooth-finished, slightly elliptical teeth and are curved to fit comfortably.

✔ **Headbands:** The old standby for keeping hair out of your face or camouflaging bang grow-out, headbands actually look best when used as *part of* a style. Look for interesting widths (very thin or very wide), interesting materials, and shades that are in line with your natural hair color — much more modern than color-coordinating your headband to your clothes. You can even make your own headbands at home by using very opaque stockings (black works best). Cut enough length off one leg and fit to head.

✔ **Hair ornaments:** Hundreds of accessories are made expressly for decorating the hair: chopstick-like picks, jeweled clips, and so on. These are great for special occasions.

✔ **Fedoras:** A very large, strong hairpin that can hold up a twist single-handedly. (These are now available in several fun colors in the U.S. from Delux; see Appendix B for contact information.)

Styling Your Hair at Home

Max Pinnell is my favorite hairstylist, and he's definitely one of the greatest hairdressers in the world. He's styled hair for everyone from Madonna to just about any Hollywood actress you could think of, not to mention all the supermodels.

Max Pinnell believes that the first step in learning how to style your hair should take place in the salon. "Ask your hairdresser to show you how to style your hair and take you through it step by step," he says. "Don't let it overwhelm you. It's like building the foundation of a house: If you take the extra time to do it right, you won't have to redo it again and again. Well-styled hair could last you three days with just touch-ups."

Part of achieving that salon look is using the right products. Pinnell is a big believer in volumizing and hair-thickening sprays. "These products are, without a doubt, the best way to get volume. They actually expand the hair shaft," he says. He also recommends leave-in conditioner to protect the hair. "It makes sense that if you put moisturizer on your skin, you should put some in your hair," Pinnell says. "Leave-in conditioner really nourishes your hair, and it's especially important if you're in the sun."

When you're using a new product at home, Pinnell advises that you go easy on the quantity and test it out a little at a time. "You can always add more, but you can't go back," he says.

Pinnell's other home-styling secret: "If you want to wear a special hairstyle for a wedding or other occasion, don't attempt something you've never tried before. Always experiment a few days early to avoid last-minute crises."

Pinnell says that the tools and products listed in Table 8-1 can help you create a variety of long and short hairstyles.

Table 8-1	What You Need to Style Your Hair
Long Hair	*Short Hair*
Round brush	Small round brush
Mason Pearson brush	Gel or mousse
Teasing brush	Volumizing spray
Rollers of your choice	Hair wax or hair cream
Volumizing spray	Hairspray
Hair cream	
Hairspray	
Laminate	

Straight hairstyles

Straight-haired women who keep it that way probably have the easiest regimen of all. With all the great products available today, it's easy to create volume and shine in even the finest straight hair. "The best way to get volume for fine, straight hair is to use volumizer — and don't be afraid to use lots of it," says stylist Max Pinnell. "It's a great way to 'dirty' your hair and give it texture."

The following sections tell you how to achieve a variety of looks for straight hair.

Very straight and shiny

I love a dead-straight hairstyle; I often do this style with my own hair. A few minutes with a blow-dryer can really boost straight hair's volume, take out kinks, and add sheen. The following steps explain how to achieve this sleek style, which is great for chin-length or longer hair that's not too layered:

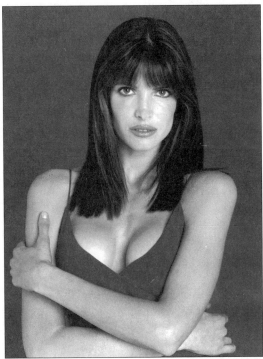

Russell James

1. **Gently comb through damp hair with a wide-tooth comb to remove tangles.**

   If you really want to boost your hair's volume, apply a volumizing or thickening product, concentrating it at the hair's roots, before blow-drying. With a spray, lift your hair section by section and spritz on the product; with a cream or gel, coat your hands with the product, flip your hair upside down, and work the product into your hair with your fingers.

2. **Blow-dry your hair, brushing it in every direction — flip it to one side, then to the other side, dry the underneath, and then flip it back again.**

   Keep doing this in every direction until your hair is almost dry. With short hair, a few seconds of blow-drying may be all you need; longer hair requires more time. If you have longer tresses, bend over so that your hair hangs upside down, and try to dry your hair evenly.

3. **Begin drying your hair straight down, using the air of the blow-dryer and a brush to create the sleekest, straightest hair possible.**

   Continue drying and brushing until your hair is completely dry. If you want your hair to be dead straight, give it a once-over with a straightening iron.

4. **Brush sleek and finish with a laminate or hair cream for sheen.**

Straight with a slight bend

This styling technique straightens your hair but leaves a bit of bend at the ends. It's good for chin-length or longer hair.

1. **Apply volumizer and shape your hair with a round brush.**

2. **Blow-dry the hair until smooth.**

   Use the technique outlined in the "Very straight and shiny" section.

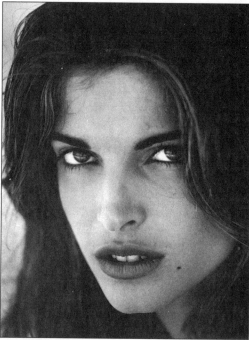

Patrick Demarchelier

3. **Set your hair in large Velcro rollers.**

   Place two rollers on the top of your head, one on each side, and one in the back.

4. **Spray the hair with aerosol hairspray. Add heat with a blow-dryer on each roller for added bend.**

5. **Wait 20 to 30 minutes and then gently remove the rollers.**

6. **Brush out your hair and add hair cream to the ends or the top if you have flyaways.**

7. **For extra height, use a teasing brush to lightly tease your hair in a 4-inch radius around the crown, and then smooth it with a brush, being careful not to flatten the height and volume that you just created.**

Sexy and tousled

Unlike the "Very straight and shiny" look, this style leaves hair wavy. It's great for any length. The following steps show you how to achieve it.

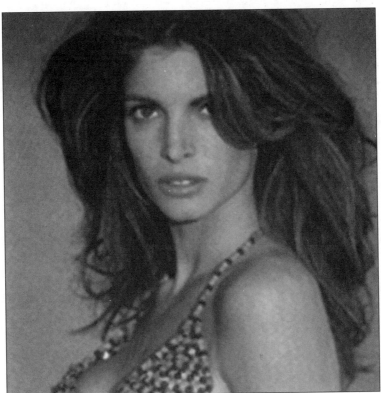

Gilles Bensimon

1. **Apply a volumizing product at the roots of your hair for lift and all over for added volume.**

2. **Using a round brush, blow-dry your hair, concentrating on drying the hair away from your face, continually brushing back and under for added volume.**

   Blow-dry your hair until it's completely dry.

3. **Use the rollers of your choice (if using steam rollers, shake out the water first), two on top, one on each side, and one in back, rolling the top ones back and the side ones under.**

   Leave the rollers in your hair for 15 to 20 minutes, or longer if you used Velcro rollers.

4. **Gently remove the rollers and allow your hair to cool for a few minutes before brushing.**

   Depending on the amount of curl you desire, you may or may not want to use a blow-dryer to loosen the curl a bit.

5. **Finish with hair cream, focusing on the ends of your hair.**

   Spray on an aerosol hairspray for extra hold if desired.

Straightening curly hair

So you've decided to fight Mother Nature and go straight? Some hair types are easier to manage than others, but it's possible to blow out any texture of hair for a straight look. The tighter the curl in your hair, however, the trickier it is to straighten it yourself while your hair is in its natural state.

Now that you've been warned, here's the secret to keeping curly hair straight: Get it 100 percent dry. If your hair is not bone-dry, it will curl up again. Start with hair that's soaking wet, and then follow these straightening steps:

1. **Lightly spray on a styling product for hold.**

2. **Use a straightening product that contains heat-activated polymers, such as Rusk Str8 or a product from John Frieda's Frizz Ease line.**

3. **Turn your head upside-down and blow-dry the extra wetness out of the hair.**

4. **Section the hair so that you can blow-dry one section at a time.**

   Hold the rest of your wet hair up with clips or elastic bands while drying.

5. **Use a strong blow-dryer and a big, round, soft brush to dry section by section, starting with the underneath sections and then working to the top layers, back to front. Wrap each section of hair around the brush, pull it taut, and blow-dry until completely dry.**

   Brush and curl the hair under while you're drying so that the hair is between the brush and the blow-dryer. Then, especially if you have hair that's one length or in long layers, you can either keep the hair curled under or toward your face as you style it, or you can use a round brush to flip the ends up for a flip look. Be careful to dry the ends while the section is wrapped around the brush.

6. **When finished (the process may take 45 minutes to an hour!), spray on a finishing product that adds shine and controls frizzy ends.**

   Look for a gel or liquid silicone-based product, such as Zotos Spa Therapy.

A couple of other thoughts on straightening:

- ✔ Use a clarifying shampoo every once in a while to strip old products from your hair; doing so helps keep the hair in better shape for straightening. Also, if you use a conditioner that's too strong and doesn't rinse out well, your hair won't respond as well. Using a protective styling spray before drying helps protect against the heat damage.

- ✔ Don't place the blow-dryer too close to your hair, or it may burn.

- ✔ There are a ton of finishing products and several anti-frizz products available. "charles worthington Results seriously shiny silkening serum" is a good line that also makes a good finisher for frizzy hair, keeping out the humidity once it's straight and keeping it straight as well as shiny. It's good to use even when you don't straighten your hair, calming down the curl and keeping flyaways under control.

- ✔ If you do a really good job of straightening your hair on a low-humidity day, it may end up almost too straight and flat. On those days, use a comb to tease your hair a tiny bit on top and add back a bit of volume.

Wavy and curly hairstyles

Women with naturally wavy or curly hair are usually the envy of women with very straight hair — and of course, women with wavy or curly hair always long for straight hair. If you think that your only option for styling your curly or wavy hair is to straighten it, get ready for a pleasant surprise. This section gives you some easy, fun, and sexy alternatives to straightening your hair. Even if you have straight hair, these techniques can give your hair a different texture.

Wavy, "beachy" hair

This hairstyle is great for women with textured or wavy hair. My hair happens to be straight, but I, of course, long for some sort of wave, so I use this technique to give my hair that wavy, "beachy," natural look.

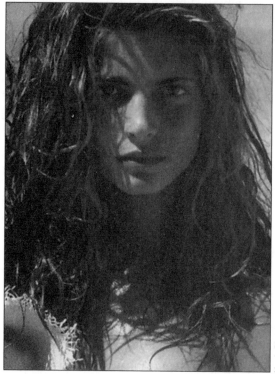

Herb Ritts

1. **Apply plenty of volumizing spray as a setting lotion and a bit of a styling cream to your hair.**

2. **If your hair is very thick, partially blow-dry it with a diffuser.**

3. **Before your hair is completely dry, separate it into small sections near your face and bigger ones toward the back of your head. Twist each section up, wrap it around your finger, lay it down on your head, and secure it with a large pin.**

   If your hair is already wavy, you can skip this step and just use a diffuser on a low setting, slowly scrunching up the hair with your hands, adding volume and wave each time you scrunch. Then spot-twist the areas that don't have as much wave as you'd like them to.

4. **Continue to dry all over your head with a diffuser until your hair is basically dry. Then let it air-dry for 20 to 30 minutes.**

5. **Take out the clips and comb through your hair with your fingers, massaging your scalp to lift the hair's roots.**

   Do not brush your hair.

6. **If desired, use hair cream or hairpins for finishing touches around your face.**

Neat curls

Natural is beautiful when it comes to curly hair. Here's how to keep it looking "undone" but still neat and pretty, while controlling the frizz.

1. **Towel-dry your hair and add volumizing spray.**

2. **Section off the hair into small, $^1/_4$-inch sections.**

3. **Twist each section of hair, wrap it around your finger, lay it down on your head, secure it with a flat clip, and allow it to air-dry.**

   If you have to dry your hair more quickly, put a diffuser on your blow-dryer and use your fingers to comb through or scrunch your hair; do not brush.

4. **If your hair looks dry on the ends or anywhere, add a touch of hair cream, squeezing it gently into the hair. Again, do not brush.**

Evening sleek

Modern, sleek hair is beautiful for evening. You can even add a barrette to the side of the hair for a more stylized look. Here's how to create this style:

1. **Apply volumizing spray to your hair and then blow-dry.**

2. **Set your hair with rollers (if using steam rollers, shake out the water first), rolling all rollers away from your face.**

   If you only have hot rollers and need to use them instead of Velcro or steam rollers, let them get warm but not hot.

3. **Take out the rollers and brush to style.**

   If your hair is too curly, you can blow-dry it out a little with a round or paddle brush.

4. **Apply hair cream on your hair's ends to keep them smooth.**

Updos

The key to an updo is to set your hair first, whether you use rollers or a round brush. "Really clean, straight hair with no bend is very difficult to work with, even for the pros," says stylist Max Pinnell. Whether your look is a sleek and sophisticated French twist or just a classic ponytail, this section gives you helpful hints to make your updos ultra-chic.

Wrapped ponytail

Nothing looks more beautiful than a simple ponytail. If you don't have time to do an updo like a French twist, a ponytail set right on your crown gives you all the lift of an updo without all the work, and it looks so pretty. Later, you can grab the end of the ponytail, roll it under, and pin it to create a gorgeous little chignon on the top of your head.

The ponytail has been around for so long for a reason: It always works — and it's better to succeed with a simple ponytail than to fail at trying something extremely complicated. You can create a ponytail with your hair totally natural, or you can blow-dry or set your hair for a more finished look. Camouflaging the elastic band with a strand of hair adds even more polish.

To create a wrapped ponytail, follow these steps:

1. **Brush all your hair into a ponytail as high or low on your head as you want it.**

2. **Secure the ponytail with an elastic.**

3. **Take a section of hair from the ponytail near the elastic (make sure that the piece is big enough to cover the band), wrap it around the elastic, and pin it under the ponytail, securing it with bobby pins.**

Breakfast at Tiffany's

This simple updo always looks chic (see page 2 of the color section) and is so easy to do yourself. Follow these steps to create this classic look:

1. **Create a ponytail near the crown of your head.**

2. **Take sections of the ponytail and curl them under, pinning them around the crown with bobby pins.**

   If you like, you can put a ribbon around the bottom of the bun for a dressier evening look. But you don't have to go so far as to wear a tiara like Audrey Hepburn does if that's not your style.

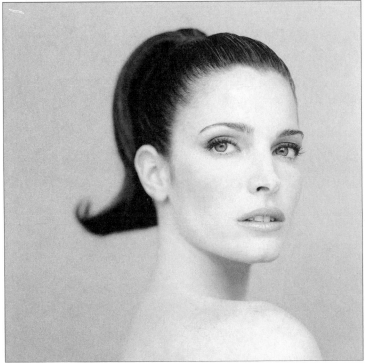

François Nars

Modern twist

This modern take on the classic French twist is one of the simplest, most elegant looks for medium-to-long hair. (The hair must be just above the shoulder or longer.) Once you master the basic moves, creating this twist is just like riding a bike — and you'll be able give yourself an updo in no time flat.

1. **Brush your hair smoothly to one side of your head.**

   Depending on whether you're left- or right-handed, brushing the hair to one side may be more comfortable for you than brushing it to the other.

2. **Using four or five bobby pins, place the pins vertically up the back of your head, slightly off center toward the side where your hair is hanging loose.**

   Fedora or Delux pins are best for this hairstyle, but they are hard to find. Try your local beauty supply store, or see Appendix B.

3. **Brush the loose hair back toward the center of your head, gripping the loose end firmly in one hand.**

4. **Turn the hair under toward your head, winding it up to your head in a tight roll from your nape.**

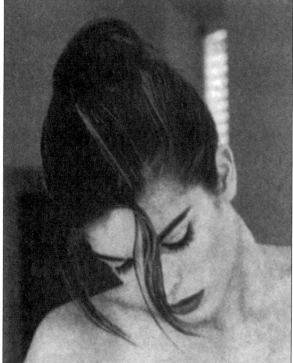

Patrick Demarchelier

5. **Twist the hair all the way to the top of your head, tuck the ends into the top of the twist, and pin the ends.**

6. **Smooth down any strays with a rattail comb, and finish with a light spritz of hairspray if needed.**

To vary the look, wind the hair tighter or more loosely, start it lower or higher on your head, or pull a few shorter strands loose near your face.

Pulling back the front

Pulling back the front of your hair is great for straight or curly hair, long or short. Here are a couple of ways to do it:

✔ Pull back the very front of the hair and pin it in the center of the head with a barrette.

✔ Pull back your bangs and pin them lightly to the side.

✔ For long hair, pull the sides all the way back, pin them at the back of the head, and let the rest of the hair hang straight.

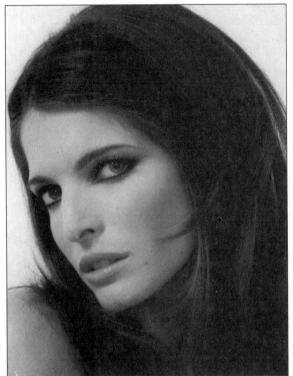

Miles Aldridge

Short hairstyles

You don't have to have long hair to create head-turning styles. With short hair, you still have plenty of options. "Hairstyling products are key for short hair more than for any other hair length," says stylist Max Pinnell. Waxes, mousses, and gels can all be used to create a variety of looks. You can use the product to bring pieces of hair onto your face or to slick the hair back away from the face. And you can even create different looks with the same product. For example, wax can be used lightly so that the hair has texture but still moves, or much heavier so that the hair becomes almost hard and very dramatic.

Here are two easy options for styling short hair:

- ✔ Use setting lotion and blow short hair out straight, blowing it forward around your face or straight back away from your face, adding hair cream for movement at the ends.

- ✔ Leave your hair wavy (if it has a natural wave). Apply hair cream and then use a diffuser, directing the air upward in places where you want your hair away from your face. You can also put a big roller at the top of your head for added height.

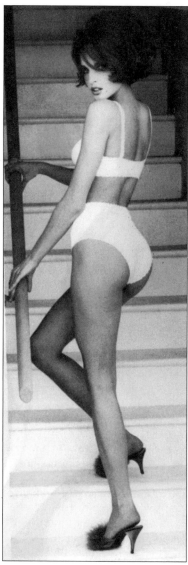

Ellen von Unwerth/A + C Anthology

Gel provides some of the best looks for short cuts. It's easy to go from an everyday bob to the slicked-back Marcel wave that was so popular in the 1920s and early 1930s. As a variation, you can skip the wave and simply comb your hair into the desired shape (behind the ears, flipped up in back) and let it set until dry. For a softer look, run a brush through your hair after it's completely dry.

The following steps help you create a sleek Marcel wave:

1. **Apply hair gel and side-part and comb your hair.**

2. **Push the hair into waves between a comb and your fingers.**

3. **Secure the waves with hairdresser's clips.**

   Leave the clips in place until the gel has set, and then gently remove them.

Falls

"You'll be amazed at how much body you can add to your hair with a simple fall," says stylist Max Pinnell, who uses falls for many of his celebrity clients. "A fall can even add up to 3 inches of length to your hair."

You can purchase falls fairly inexpensively at specialty stores. Pinnell suggests that you check with your stylist for a store in your area. Then it's simply a matter of matching the color to your own hair.

"You can even take the fall in to your stylist to cut so that it matches the length of your hair," Pinnell says. "The stylist can show you how to put it in and blend it."

Falls are wonderful for updos, especially if you don't have enough hair to make such styles work. Some falls are made to be swept up, Pinnell says, and others are wonderful for creating a thick ponytail or making a nice chignon.

To insert a fall, lift up your hair and pin the fall about an inch down from the crown of your head. Smooth your natural hair over it, and you're ready to go.

Chapter 9
Hair Q & A

The only predictable thing about hair is that it's usually every woman's pet peeve. No matter how skilled you are with styling or how many times you've colored your hair at home, you always face some unexpected trauma. Fear not — help is here for the most common hair dilemmas and disasters.

Haircuts

This section answers some common questions about hair-cutting and styling.

I have a cowlick at my hairline. What can I do to fix it?

You have two choices: fight it or work with it. You can tame most cowlicks by using a blow-dryer or roller to redirect the hair against its natural growth pattern. You can coax more-severe cowlicks to lie down by spot-perming — something only a pro should attempt. Bangs are especially difficult when a cowlick's at work: You need a fringe with sufficient weight and length to outmuscle the cowlick after it's styled in place. Styling gel is helpful.

A very pronounced cowlick is tough to fight successfully, so unless you're ready to reshape your entire hairline through electrolysis à la Rita Hayworth, you should work with your stylist to find a style that incorporates the cowlick as a feature of the cut. If you let it determine where your hair "breaks" and you keep its pattern of growth, you won't have a daily battle on your hands. In fact, you may come to appreciate your cowlick as a unique and individual aspect of your appearance.

How do I know the best place to part my hair?

There's no such thing as a "best" place. If you have a long face or a pronounced nose, avoid center parts. Otherwise, where you part your hair can depend on where you have cowlicks or which side of your face you want to flatter. Experiment and go with what *you* think looks best.

I want to grow out my hair, but I fear the in-between stage — especially with my bangs. Any advice?

The best way to get through an awkward growing-out phase? "I'm a big believer in just letting it go," says stylist Max Pinnell. "Once you start cleaning it up and trying to compromise with some kind of in-between style, you usually end up with a no-style style that's worse than if you did nothing at all. Just let it be a little messy and imperfect." That's not to say that you should abandon trims altogether, however. They're still a must, especially if you're growing out very damaged, overprocessed hair.

Bang grow-out can be particularly frustrating, but a little pre-grow-out cut can help here, too. Have your stylist add a few long, angled layers near your face to take the edge off your bangs and help them blend in as they grow. And don't forget that headbands, barrettes, styling products, and ponytails are all great ways to ease the transition and keep stray strands out of your way.

What do I do if I hate my haircut?

Granted, some cuts are a cut above others. I'm not talking about those minor differences here; I'm talking about a bad cut that sends you running for cover. For example, I have very thick hair. Everybody wants to layer it, which is a total disaster because it only makes my hair thicker and "piecey." It doesn't look soft, it's more difficult to style, and it takes forever to grow out. Here's how to handle a cut that you're unhappy with:

- ✔ **If a pro did it:** By all means, ask that it be fixed. If the problem is over-layering or not enough length, your only option is to let it grow.
- ✔ **If you did it:** Don't make a bad situation worse — go to a pro.

Chemical Processes

Chemical processing can be the most confusing — and most abusing — part of hair care. This section addresses common dilemmas that I often hear women discuss.

The ends of my hair are much darker than my roots. How do I fix this problem?

Women who color their hair at home commonly have this problem. According to colorist Bryan Thomson, "What you're seeing is color build-up from dragging the hair color all the way through your hair every time you use it. The ends just keep getting darker and darker until they're oversaturated." Unless you're using hair color for the very first time — even if you've switched product types or colors — you should apply the product to new growth *only* and work it through to hair ends for only a few minutes before rinsing it out. Because the ends are the oldest part of your hair, and therefore the most damaged and porous, they absorb color more quickly than the healthier hair at root level.

When you color your hair the next time, follow the manufacturer's instructions for a retouch application and see whether that helps even things out. If you're still stuck with a two-tone 'do, see a pro.

When I color my hair, my gray hairs never seem to take the color properly. Am I doing something wrong?

The first thing you need to check is the type of hair color formula you've been using. Labels can be confusing, and you may have picked up a product that isn't capable of fully covering gray. (See Chapter 7 for information about the different formulas and their best uses.) For complete, lasting gray coverage, you need to use a *permanent* formula and leave it on long enough to penetrate thoroughly. (Covering your hair with a plastic cap to trap body heat can also help color absorb.)

You may also be responding to the fact that hair color looks lighter over your gray strands than on your naturally pigmented hair. As Chapter 7 recommends, it's always better to choose a hair color shade that's a few shades lighter than your real color. That, of course, shows up even lighter when applied over gray strands. Unless you're getting a very marked contrast, this is actually a *good* thing: The mixture of shades gives the hair added highlights and dimension. What you *don't* want to do is switch to a darker shade or leave the product on too long, hoping for greater coverage — you'll wind up with color that looks flat.

Some gray hair is just extremely resistant to hair color, and products formulated for home use may not be strong enough for the job. If permanent home hair color is not giving you the coverage you want, see a professional colorist.

How do I remedy a bad perm?

Playing with chemicals is a tricky process. Mistakes are not uncommon, especially with do-it-yourself home perms. Frizziness and breakage are signs that the rods were wrapped too tightly; uneven curl comes from uneven tension on the rods or uneven application or rinsing of solutions or neutralizer. Here's how to remedy the problem:

- ✔ **If you did it:** Immediately wash and deep-condition your hair to loosen the curl, using heat if possible; then blow-dry it straight. Correct frizziness by relaxing the hair with more perm solution (do not roll it again), but be careful: You may end up with damage.

- ✔ **If a pro did it:** Have the salon fix it immediately if possible; otherwise, wait a week to redo the perm and condition well in the meantime. Of course, you should have the salon fix the problem only if you feel confident in the technician's abilities. If you don't, get the name of the product that was used and find another hair technician to redo your perm.

How many chemical processes can you do without destroying your hair? And how long should you wait between processes?

It really depends on your hair's health and the types of processes you want to have done, but no hair is invincible when faced with repeated chemical services. In general, the harshest processes — perming, straightening, and permanent hair coloring — should be done to the hair only once, reapplied only to new growth, and rarely, if ever, used in combination (in the case of straightening, *never*). If your hair's in good condition, a few days to a week between services (say, perming and then coloring) or reapplication of the same process (as in color correction) should be sufficient. Alhough the damage is done and your hair won't "recover" in the interim, you'll be able to get in a few good conditioning treatments to help counteract your hair's new, more porous state.

Nothing I do makes my hair look better — no cut, no color, no perm. How can I figure out what's wrong?

Dozens of factors affect your hair's appearance. Some (such as using the wrong products) are easily fixed; others (such as poor health) are more difficult to overcome. The best approach to identifying the problem is to enlist the help of your stylist *and* your doctor. Your stylist can tell you whether the products or styling techniques you're using are ineffective or even damaging; your physician can rule out health conditions that may be contributing to the poor appearance of your hair.

You may also want to consult a *trichologist* — a professional who analyzes the hair and scalp to determine possible causes of hair problems. Some salons have trichologists on staff or can refer you to companies, including J. F. Lazartigue, Redken, and Philip Kingsley, that do this type of analysis (see Appendix B for contact information). Be warned that a degree of skepticism surrounds trichology, and that the products manufactured and recommended by such companies are not cheap, but if you're at the end of your rope, you may find it worth the expense if you get good results.

In the meantime, look over the following list of common hair-wreckers. Self-diagnose the damage that you may be inflicting upon yourself and pinpoint areas to discuss with your stylist and physician:

- ✔ **Processing and styling:** Perming, chemical straightening, repeated or harsh hair coloring, overbrushing, excessive and/or repeated heat from blow-dryers, curling irons, pressing irons, and other heat-styling appliances

- ✔ **Environment:** Sun, pollution, chlorine, salt water, wind, trace elements and minerals in tap water, too much or too little humidity

- ✔ **Medications:** Birth control pills, antibiotics, amphetamines, tranquilizers or sedatives, thyroid drugs, cortisones

> ✔ **Health and heredity:** Stress, poor diet, anorexia or bulimia, chronic or catastrophic illness, hormone fluctuations or imbalances, genetic predispositions

Hair Emergencies

Before you give up on your hair altogether and throw on a baseball cap, read through this section — you may find the remedy for your particular hair emergency.

I'm only 24 and my hair's already going gray. Is there any way to reverse this?

Premature graying is usually caused by heredity, but it can also be a sign of such health problems as diabetes, thyroid disorders, and anemia. Discuss your concerns with your physician, especially if such conditions run in your family, and ask for a comprehensive check-up to rule out a physiological reason for the change. If a health-related factor is causing you to go gray, you may see pigmentation return after your body's in a healthier state.

Stress also may be a factor: It depletes the body of B vitamins, which some studies have shown to help restore pigment to graying hair when taken in large doses. However, it's more likely that you're perfectly healthy and that early graying simply runs in your family — and that, unfortunately, is not reversible. If the silver strands bother you, see Chapter 7 for tips on coloring your hair.

My hair is falling out. What should I do?

Discovering the cause of hair loss is not always easy. A variety of factors cause the problem, ranging from stress that results in hormonal changes, poor diet, hormones, anemia, eating disorders, medications, and health problems (including illness and surgery) to excessive exercise that affects the body's hormones.

The first thing you must determine is whether your hair is falling out from the root or breaking off at some point along the shaft. Examine a few fallen hairs closely: Are they about as long as the other hairs on your head? Do they show a definite root end? Or are they smaller pieces with frayed, broken ends?

✔ **Hair breaking off:** If your hair is breaking off in pieces, it's clear that your hair is seriously damaged. The only question is, what caused the damage? A stylist can point out whether the problem is from color or styling, too much heat and handling, overprocessing, or something more serious. Hair breakage can also result from an eating disorder; environmental damage from sun, water, and wind; overly tight ponytails or braids; uncovered elastics; accessories with teeth (headbands and barrettes); or hats.

The usual solution for hair breakage is to deep-condition regularly, treat your hair very gently, limit blow-drying and mechanical styling, and trim off as much of the damaged hair as possible.

✔ **Hair thinning/receding:** Losing some hair every day, as old hair is replaced by new hair, is perfectly normal. What's more troubling is the thinning and receding of hair caused by new hair that is thinner in diameter. The result? Hair that gradually loses body and volume. Many things cause hair thinning and receding, including *traction alopecia,* which is commonly found in African-Americans and develops due to usage of pulling and straightening methods; and *alopecia areata,* which causes hair to fall out in patches and may be caused by stress. (A dermatologist can prescribe a course of medication that can help rectify this problem.)

It's not uncommon to see a gradual overall thinning with age. By age 40, everyone has hair that's thinner than it was at age 25. Other than the typical aging process, thinning hair can be the result of your own hormones changing or hormonal supplements that you're taking by prescription. Women do experience male-pattern baldness (caused by hormone and thyroid problems), but all-over thinning is more common.

In any case, it's a good idea to see a dermatologist so that he or she can determine what's happening in your particular case. With genetic hair loss, a combination of hormone therapy and topical drugs can get good regrowth results. Your gynecologist and/or dermatologist are good resources for information and may refer you to an *endocrinologist,* a specialist in hormones.

✔ **Hair falling out in clumps:** Medical conditions can cause hair loss. Post-partum women can shed up to 30 percent of their hair. In addition, cancer, anorexia, improper nutrition, ringworm, and alopecia all cause hair loss. In any of these cases, please take your health seriously and see a doctor.

Pregnancy and post-pregnancy hair

During pregnancy, with estrogen in overdrive, many women find that their hair is thicker, sturdier, and shinier than ever. After the baby is born, however, hormonal changes may produce the opposite results: hair that's dry and brittle, and hair that sheds. The reason? Hormonal changes during pregnancy result in the scalp producing less sebum, which means that hair is less weighed down and therefore feels thicker. In fact, your hair's growth phase is extended during pregnancy due to the hormones that are released, so it can grow longer.

About half of women experience post-partum alopecia (or hair loss), which can happen up to three months after delivery and can last about three months. The heavy hair loss occurs because the level of estrogen is returning to normal. The hair that would have reached the end of its extended growth phase during pregnancy reverts to its old cycle and falls out instead.

The good news: Your hair will grow back. Until then, your hair loss will take its natural course. Just be patient and wait it out. While waiting for your hair to return to its pre-pregnancy state, treat your hair and scalp to protein moisturizing shampoos and conditioners and trim it as often as possible.

My hair is thinning more and more as I age. How can I make it look thicker?

Hair *does* naturally thin out over time — in both diameter and number of hairs in total — but first you want to determine, with your doctor, whether your thinning hair is simply a matter of age, or whether other factors are at work. To prevent further fallout and help regrow some of what was lost, you may be a candidate for Rogaine (minoxidil), which is now available without a prescription in the United States. "Rogaine promotes hair growth, but it can also act as a setting lotion to make the hair thicker," says stylist Howard Fuglar.

Fuglar is also an advocate of applying cream to the ends of hair and using a thickening cream before blow-drying to give body. He advises avoiding products containing alcohol because alcohol makes hair "crisp." Another idea: Temporary hair colors to cover thinning areas. With a cotton ball, dab a shade that matches your hair onto your scalp to hide sparse, shiny areas.

How do I handle my hair on a very humid day?

Hair loses its shape when there's too much moisture in the air. Healthy hair can absorb its own weight in water and swell almost 15 percent in diameter — bad news if you just spent 20 minutes smoothing everything down with your blow-dryer. How to short-circuit humidity's damaging effects? Style your hair straight and then use a product that contains a silicone or a similar ingredient plus a moisturizer in an emulsion form. In general, a creamy product is more effective than a clear, transparent product at achieving manageable hair that stays manageable in humid weather.

How can I fix my hair fast?

Hat head. A bad day at the salon. Sprinting for a cab in July. A blast of cold wind on a winter's day. Any of these can get you off to a Bad Hair Day. Following are a few fast fixes for these minor hair traumas:

- ✔ **Carry volumizer spray.** If you have straight or fine hair that is out of place or has gone flat due to bad weather, volumizer is a great fix. Just flip your hair over, brush it while it's flipped, spray the roots with volumizer, dry it with a hand dryer, and then brush it back. (Don't pull the roots; just brush the ends.) You'll have a head of full hair.

- ✔ **Carry texturizing balm.** For curly hair, run a little texturizing balm through your hair to take away the frizzies caused by humidity, rain, or perspiration.

- ✔ **Carry a hair moisturizer or hair cream.** A little hair cream is great for taming ends or flyaways.

- ✔ **Carry barrettes or bands.** Pulling your hair back is always a solution if it feels grimy and you can't wash it. After you pull it up, pull a few pieces down around your face if you think that it looks too harsh. A ponytail is always a nice, simple style that makes you look pulled-together. (See Chapter 8 for step-by-step information about these hairstyles.)

I swim several days a week for exercise, but it's killing my hair and turning it green. What can I do?

Proper care both before *and* after you hit the pool safeguards your hair's health and color. Prior to your swim, coat your hair with conditioner and then tuck everything securely under a close-fitting swim cap or two.

Afterwards, rinse your hair immediately and thoroughly with fresh water. To counteract chlorine's drying effects, use an intensive conditioner after shampooing and give your hair an occasional deep-conditioning treatment (see Chapter 5 for details) when it's feeling extra dry.

Regular use of a clarifying shampoo or special build-up remover — especially for blondes — helps get rid of unwanted deposits. "If you've already got really bad build-up, put a clarifier on your hair and then a plastic shower cap and leave it on for about 20 minutes," advises colorist Bryan Thomson. "It will pull out that greenish tinge and bring your color back to normal."

Ever since I moved to a new area, my hair has looked awful. Could it be the water?

When I travel, my hair looks different everywhere I go — and yes, it's because of the water. In Paris, my hair's always terrible. When I was a child, my hair turned red from the iron in our tap water. The trace metals and minerals that some water contains can leave a definite color tinge in your hair, prevent shampoos from lathering well, and leave deposits along the hair shaft that make styling more difficult.

If you have hard water, you can do a number of things to counteract its hair-dulling effects: At home, install a water softener or buy a filter for your shower head. When traveling, use a clarifying shampoo or find a shampoo that's made to work in hard water.

Hair Care

You may wonder how to make your hair look and feel healthier. This section answers a few questions relating to hair health and care.

Do vitamins or other dietary supplements help the hair?

The only vitamin known to have a beneficial effect when applied to the hair is *panthenol,* a derivative of vitamin B (see Chapter 5 for more information). The current craze in skin care for free-radical fighters such as vitamins A, C, and E has led to their being included in many hair care products, but there's no conclusive proof that they have an antioxidant effect on the hair. (Oxidization is one reason that hair color fades or turns brassy.)

As for vitamins that you can take internally, they're not really necessary if you eat a balanced diet. However, if your eating habits are sporadic or less than healthy, a good multivitamin supplement that includes vitamin B complex, vitamin A, and key minerals such as calcium and magnesium will help make up for deficiencies that may affect your hair.

How can I make my hair look shinier?

Shine is a matter of how evenly light reflects off the hair's surface. Some hair types have a head start when it comes to shine: The cuticle of straight and wavy hair naturally forms a smooth, even surface along the hair shaft, resulting in a glossy appearance. Because the surface of curly or kinky hair is less even, it reflects light irregularly, resulting in more of a sheen than the true glass-like shine that straighter hair can have.

You can trace dulled hair to overconditioning, product build-up, and hard water, but the real shine-destroyer is damage from chemical processes, overmanipulation, or excessive heat-styling. The more you chip away at the cuticle with such abuse, the less even the hair's surface becomes, until it reflects light poorly and develops a lackluster appearance. To restore hair's shine, limiting such abuse is priority number one. You can also take a number of steps to get the gloss back:

✔ Wash your hair with a clarifying shampoo and follow with conditioner only where (and if) needed. "Most women use too much conditioner, and that can dull the hair," says stylist and salon owner Frederic Fekkai. "You don't need it on your scalp — it should be from the middle of the shaft to the ends *only*. Comb it through and rinse it very, very well." He also recommends finishing with a cool-water rinse or acidic finishing rinse to close the hair's cuticle.

✔ Alternate shampoos regularly to keep build-up at bay, and invest in a shower-head water filter if you suspect that your area's tap water has a high mineral content.

✔ Apply a small amount of silicone-based styling product to your hair — wet or dry, depending on the product you're using — distributing it sparingly and evenly throughout the hair. Avoid the scalp and roots, or you may end up with hair that feels greasy.

✔ Blow-drying is an effective way to boost the shine of straight and wavy styles because high heat helps flatten the cuticle. The trick is to use a very hot setting and fast-moving air, directing the air flow from roots to ends, and using a natural-bristle brush to help smooth the cuticle in the direction of growth. "When you're done blow-drying, finish with cool air," Fekkai recommends. "It makes the hair very shiny and beautiful."

✔ Hair color can also help revive shine in dull hair, especially if it's been overlightened. Use a gentle semi- or demipermanent formula if you're coloring at home, or "go to the colorist and get a gloss or reverse highlights," recommends Fekkai. "Reverse highlights will put some contrast back in your hair, and because you're putting color back in, not taking it out, your hair will be less porous and get more shine."

What's the best way to get rid of static and flyaways?

Because static occurs when the air around you is dry, the ideal way to prevent the problem is to use a humidifier to boost the air's moisture (which is great for keeping your skin supple, too). But because it's impossible to control your personal climate 24 hours a day, you can also try spritzing your hairbrush with hairspray (or an anti-static spray) and then brushing through, or applying a little leave-in conditioner, styling cream, or silicone-based product to help smooth down flyaways.

I have straight hair that's very fine and flat. How can I build up body?

Start by keeping your hair very, very clean. Anything that leaves a coating on the hair shaft — conditioners, styling products, even your scalp's natural oils — weighs it down and can give your hair a flat look. Consider using body-boosting or volumizing shampoos that contain humectants such as glycerin, hyaluronic acid, or sorbitol. These ingredients attract water to the hair shaft, which swells it, giving you a feeling of greater fullness. Use conditioner only on your hair ends and only if needed; leave-in conditioners or detanglers are good, lightweight options for fine hair. Give your roots a boost with mousse or volumizing spray before blow-drying, and dry your hair upside-down — the anti-gravity position helps build fullness and lift.

Color can also make a real difference in making your hair appear fuller. Says salon owner and stylist Frederic Fekkai, "I often suggest highlights to my clients with fine hair — or lowlights for someone who wouldn't look good going lighter. It adds contrast, coats the hair, and gives the body and texture the hair needs."

Finally, you need a great haircut that makes the most of your hair. Remember, the less weight, the better, so stick with styles that are shoulder length or above.

Looking Great

Whether you're planning for a big day like a wedding or you just want to look your best from day to day, this section can help.

How can I be sure that my hair looks great for my wedding day?

As with everything wedding-related, the key is to *plan ahead*. First, consider the general look you want. If you want your hair to be as long as possible and you have half a year to get there, for example, you'll need to plan for a serious grow-out phase. If you're looking to make a change with cut and color, work with your stylist as far in advance as you can to find a new direction that you're comfortable with.

Your hairstylist will never be more valuable to you than when you're planning your wedding look. He or she can guide you through all the decisions you never realized had to be made. Even if your ceremony is very casual or you're just not the type to fuss over your hair, enlisting a pro's help *is* a good idea — if only to get some special do-it-yourself styling tips. Going to a pro for wedding-day styling is a rare treat that also gives you a little pampering on what's sure to be a very hectic day. Keep these tips in mind as you and your stylist work on your look:

- ✔ You want a style that's still "you," yet works with all the other variables of your wedding day: the ceremony's season and time of day, the style and formality of your dress, and the headpiece you'll be wearing — veil, hat, floral wreath, or tiara, for example. You'll need your headpiece at least a few weeks before the ceremony for practice purposes in the salon.

- ✔ For comfort and ease of movement, most brides either partially or totally remove their headpieces for the reception. Make sure that your style will look good in both situations, and that the headpiece can be removed or altered without destroying your style.

- ✔ Visualize yourself at the reception, and plan for a style that's in tune with *what* you'll be doing and *where* you'll be doing it. If you plan to spend hours whirling around the dance floor or will be outdoors on a breezy bay, a towering updo won't last for long.

- ✔ Because most weddings take place on weekends, book your stylist as soon as you settle on a date. Bridal 'dos can be time-intensive, taking up several appointments' worth of time in the salon (or at your home), and the stylist needs to arrange his or her schedule accordingly. Be sure to call the day before to confirm — this is one appointment you can't afford to miss.

✔ Have any permanent chemical processes — coloring, perming, or straightening — done about two weeks before the big day. That way, you'll have plenty of time to get used to your new hair and can correct any problems without racing against the clock.

✔ Don't do anything radically different or elaborate, such as suddenly going very short or submitting to an overblown updo. You won't feel like yourself — not exactly the best frame of mind to be in on your wedding day.

✔ If your hair is left loose, resist the urge to shellac it into place with hairspray. You don't want to have to keep adjusting it during the ceremony and reception, but stiff hair is never flattering. Plan with your stylist beforehand so that you find a style that you won't have to fuss with, but that's still soft and pretty.

How can I keep my hair looking great all day?

It all starts with the right hairstyle. Anything elaborate or at odds with your hair's natural tendencies is difficult to maintain; a simple style that works *with* your hair, not against it, makes maintenance easier.

The other key to keeping hair looking good is to take the time to style it properly. "It's like building the foundation of a house," says stylist Max Pinnell. "If you want it to last, you can't rush it, and you need to use the right techniques. Say you're blow-drying your hair — you have to work section by section, using the right brush and some kind of styling product like a lotion or volumizer." (See Chapter 8 for pro styling tips.) Taking more time on your hair actually *saves* you time in the long run, according to Pinnell. "If you spend, say, a half-hour to style your hair right from the start, you won't have to restyle it during the day — and it could even last you *three* days. All you'll have to do is touch it up in the morning, and you're ready to go."

Part III
Makeup

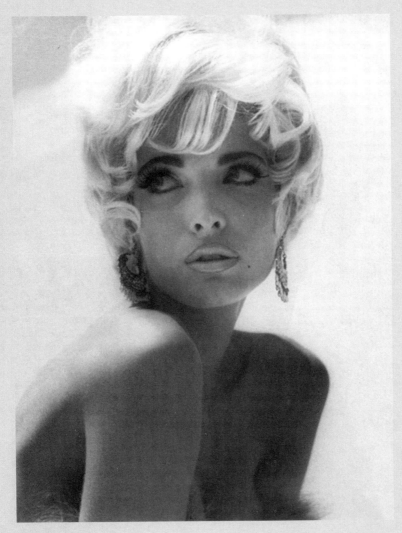

In this part . . .

Makeup has always been many things to many different kinds of people. Over the centuries, it's been used to prepare the body for religious rituals, regarded as a sign of one's social standing, and even considered evidence of a lack of morals. So let me say two things up front: You do not *have* to wear makeup, but you have no reason to feel vain or frivolous for being interested in wearing makeup. Truth is, humans have adorned themselves with color since time began.

Makeup exists to give you confidence, to smooth over the things that you'd rather hide, and to play up the things that you like. You can wear a little, or you can wear a lot. It's up to you.

This part gives you all the vital information on makeup — the formulas, the colors, and the best application methods.

Chapter 10

Finding Your Style

. . . .

In This Chapter

▶ Defining your own makeup style

▶ Putting your best face forward at any age

. . . .

*I*t took me a long time to learn about makeup. When I was about 13 years old, my mother would put a little makeup on me for special occasions — a little blush, a little mascara, a little pink lipstick, and that was *it*. She finally gave in and bought me a soft-colored blush that I was allowed to wear every day and a Bonne Bell Lip Smacker. Because that was all I had, I got everything I could out of it. I put the Lip Smacker on my eyelids because I liked them to look shiny, and I used loads of blush so I'd look like I had just taken the sun.

When I was 14, I won the regional Look of the Year contest in San Diego, California. One of the things they gave me as a winner was a free enrollment at the John Casablancas School of Modeling. I had two more contests to go — in New York, and then in Acapulco — so the courses were to prepare me for the next two competitions. They taught me to do a very heavy makeup using lots of pancake base and cheek contour — and I was 14 years old! Putting on all that makeup just wasn't me, but I was pretty naive and didn't know any better.

Since then, I've worked with some of the greatest makeup artists in the world. I've learned to love makeup for what it can do for my face, and hate it when it becomes a mask. Over the years, I've realized that *I* know my face and what looks good on it better than anyone else. All the best makeup artists agree: You have to trust yourself.

In this chapter, I'll help you define your own personal style. Whether you prefer a natural look or a more expressive approach, you'll find guidelines that help you find your best look — no matter what your age.

Basic Makeup Philosophies

Makeup can be a strong style statement. It's a reflection of who you are and how you feel. And sometimes it's more complicated than "natural is best." Makeup has to go with your personality, the way you dress — even your mood. From the moment you make your first fumbling attempts with color, you're defining your own makeup style. With time — and lots of trial and error — you get to know your comfort level with makeup and the unique quirks of your face.

Although no two women have the exact same approach, two basic philosophies of makeup *do* seem to hold true. You may fall squarely into one category or the other, or you may decide to jump back and forth at will, like I do.

✔ **Second nature:** You use makeup to enhance your eyes, cheeks, and lips and to even out your skin tone. Whether you do this with a little concealer, lip gloss, and blush, or you enhance a little bit of everything, you're not necessarily making a statement with your makeup. You just want to look natural. For you, makeup is for looking fresher, prettier, and more pulled-together.

Icons of this makeup style include Julie Christie, Katharine Hepburn, Grace Kelly, and Katharine Ross.

✔ **Making a statement:** You use makeup as a means of self-expression. You're not afraid to be bold or different; you like to play with color and make a statement with your eyes or lips. Whether you wear a bright red lip with a little bit of eyeliner like Marilyn, or you do a smoky eye with a pale lip like Bardot, you're expressing yourself or your mood.

Icons of this makeup style include Brigitte Bardot, Sophia Loren, Marilyn Monroe, and Marlene Dietrich.

Keeping It Personal

Getting a mental image of makeup looks from the past is very easy. If I say 1920s, you immediately see a flapper with cupid's bow lips and kohled eyes; the 1960s was thick liquid liner, false eyelashes, and pale pink lips. Okay, how about *now*? Right now — what's the look? You can't come up with just one image, can you? That's because women don't accept the cookie-cutter approach to makeup anymore. Now, the "look" is about looking like yourself and embracing your individuality.

Playing around with new trends and past classics is fun, but don't get too caught up in them. There's only one foolproof way to be sure that you're wearing the right makeup: Always use yourself as the starting point — your skin tone, your preferences, your personality. After you establish your *own* makeup style, simply vary your look to fit the following factors:

- ✔ **Your mood:** Your style may be understated most of the time, but sometimes your internal glamour-puss begs for attention. Indulge!

- ✔ **Your age:** A 15-year-old's fuchsia lip gloss looks ridiculous on a 55-year-old. See "Looking Great at Any Age" later in this chapter for tips on age-proofing your makeup application.

- ✔ **The weather:** A full face of matte makeup looks, and feels, very artificial in summer's intense light and heat. The basic rule: Less makeup and lighter textures are better in summer (or in hot climates), and more coverage and richer formulas work better in winter.

- ✔ **Your destination:** You wouldn't wear the same clothes to the office, a black-tie event, and a family picnic — nor should you wear the same makeup. Tailor it accordingly.

- ✔ **Your skin condition:** When you have a Bad Skin Day, boost coverage to even things out; when skin's looking great, you may decide to skip makeup altogether.

- ✔ **The time of day:** Nighttime's artificial light is not as strong as natural daylight, so go for deeper tones and more intensity in your evening makeup. If you usually follow the second nature philosophy, evening may be a good time for you to make a statement.

- ✔ **Changes to your coloring:** If you get a tan or a radically different hair color, you need to alter your makeup to go with the change.

- ✔ **Your comfort level:** If you're uneasy about wearing makeup or unsure of your application skills, take small steps. Practice and stick with the basics 'til you have it down pat, and *then* try the more complicated moves.

Keep in mind that makeup *needs* to change to stay modern. Re-evaluate your look often, and don't be afraid to try new things (see "Getting Out of a Rut" in Chapter 11 for more info). For inspiration, check out the full-color Makeup Workbook to see lots of great makeup looks — complete with easy application how-tos.

Looking Great at Any Age

You should always be aware of how your looks evolve over time — and how to accommodate those changes with makeup. Of course, every woman is an individual, with a face that changes in different ways and at different rates, so regard these numbers as a guide.

Teens

Once you finally get the go-ahead to wear makeup, you may be tempted to pile it on. Don't — you'll only look like a little girl playing in her mother's makeup bag, which is the last thing you want. But that doesn't mean you can't have fun — in fact, I encourage you to experiment. This is the only time in your life when green mascara and sparkly lipstick are going to be passable, so get it out of your system now!

- ✔ The biggest favor you can do for your skin at this age: Wear sunscreen every day (see Chapter 1 for more info about sun and skin).

- ✔ Young skin tends to be oily and acne-prone, but piling on powder and foundation is not the solution — you'll look like you're wearing a mask, and you may even clog your pores and make things worse. Use concealer to cover the occasional blemish (see Chapter 14 for how-tos), a very lightweight oil-free foundation to even out larger areas (*only* if you need to), and a little powder to cut shine. If acne or breakouts are common occurrences, don't just cover it up — clear it up with the help of a dermatologist. (See Chapter 3 to figure out when you really need a doctor — and how to find one.)

- ✔ If you want to play with funky colors, limit them to one area of the face — eyes *or* lips, not both.

- ✔ If you want to use shine, sparkle, or iridescence, apply it with a light touch. These finishes look great on young skin, but you don't want to overdo it.

- ✔ Many girls begin tweezing their brows around this age — *please* use restraint. Although a radically reshaped brow may strike you as more "adult," it really looks overdone, especially on a young face. Have an adult or a professional help you until you get the hang of it, follow the guidelines for a basic cleanup in Chapter 13, or check out Chapter 13's list of alternatives to brow-shaping.

- ✔ If you have braces, wear a tinted lip balm or a very light, sheer lipstick for color. Anything too dark draws attention to your mouth and may wind up on the wires.

Twenties

You may be pressed for time in your twenties, but that's not to say that you're not interested in how you look. This is a great time to experiment, either in a way that looks very natural or by making a statement with your makeup; experimenting helps you figure out who you are and what you like.

You also need to develop a few basic makeup moves that you can rely on: perfecting your skin, enhancing your eyes, and creating a great lip.

- ✔ Use sunscreen on your face every day.

- ✔ Your skin is probably not as oily as it once was, but acne may flare up. Opt for a lightweight, oil-free foundation when you want more coverage, or just spot on concealer with a brush where you need it to take down redness.

- ✔ Less sleep can mean undereye darkness and puffiness. Use a cooling eye gel to reduce the puffiness, and then apply concealer five to ten minutes later to even out eye-area darkness (find out how in Chapter 14). You'll immediately look more rested.

- ✔ As you reach your later twenties, use a light foundation or loose powder to perfect your skin's color and texture.

- ✔ When you're under time constraints, stick to a natural look; keep it simple. Neutral shades apply quickly, forgive less-than-precise placement, and help you look pulled-together fast.

- ✔ If you're going out, pull out all the stops and indulge your inner diva. Play with color, taking your time to figure out what looks best. If you *don't* have plans for the evening, pull out your makeup bag anyway and try some new things. This is a great way to perfect your makeup application skills and may just help you find a great new look.

Thirties

You know who you are, what you like, and what looks good on you. But you may start to notice unevenness in your skin tone and a few lines creeping in around your eyes. Now is the time to pay closer attention to *texture* and *technique:* Make sure that you apply your makeup formulas smoothly and evenly over your skin, and that you place and blend color with precision.

- ✔ Wear sunscreen daily.

- ✔ Instead of taking the sun, use powder or cream bronzer to give areas of your face a sun-kissed glow.

- ✔ On days when your skin doesn't look its best, a very thin, well-blended layer of foundation evens your skin tone and boosts your confidence.

- ✔ If you notice that your skin is feeling drier, especially in winter or dry climates, you need to add more moisture to your skin. Begin wearing moisturizer under your makeup if you aren't already, or opt for makeup with moisturizing properties.

- ✔ In your mid- to late thirties, you may want to use a creamier, more moisturizing foundation formula.

✔ Thinner, drier eye-area skin is more prone to makeup creasing. Make sure that the area is well-moisturized before concealer goes on. To reduce puffiness, apply a cooling eye gel five to ten minutes before applying concealer.

Forties

The forties are a beautiful, sexy age for women; don't let signs of aging shock you or make you feel less youthful and vibrant. Your skin may be drier and less elastic than it once was, and facial lines may be more abundant and pronounced. Changes in skin tone also become more apparent — your natural skin and lip pigment may fade and become uneven, so be sure to wear blush and lip color to prevent a pale, washed-out look.

✔ Don't go after a dark tan. A dark tan doesn't make you look younger; it only dries out the skin and makes facial lines more obvious. To add a bit of color to your face, use powder or cream bronzer — avoid self-tanning lotions, which usually only make your skin look orange. And remember to use sunscreen every day.

✔ Use a moisturizing foundation with light-refracting ingredients to help restore a supple look and feel to the skin and play down facial lines. To keep makeup in place, set it with a silky, finely milled face powder.

✔ Be careful with shimmery products, especially on your eyes; they tend to collect in creases.

✔ Use a volumizing mascara to help bring lushness back to lashes that may seem thinner and less abundant, but don't overdo it. Use an eyelash comb to comb through lashes after applying a thick coat of mascara.

✔ Take extra care to moisturize under makeup if you're using powder blusher, because powder products tend to "sit" on drier skin. Creamy blushers are a great option for creating a healthy, radiant glow. On your eyes, however, creamy pencils and shadows can collect in creases. Set their color with powder, or just use powder color instead.

✔ Make sure to apply moisturizer to your undereye area before applying concealer. Use a heavier eye cream in the evening than you do during the day; you need all the moisture that you can get around your eyes.

✔ Touch up lipstick throughout the day, no matter how busy or tired you may feel. It will help keep you looking fresh and finished.

✔ Use liner and/or a dusting of powder to keep color in place if lipstick feathering is a problem. (See Chapter 14 for application techniques.)

Fifties

At this stage in your life, you see lots of changes in your skin. It may get lighter, so this is a good time to focus on hair color — the right color can really brighten up your face. Your skin tone may have faded, but don't make the classic mistake of wearing a pink-toned foundation. Concentrate on giving an even, natural-looking finish to the skin, gentle definition to the eyes, and color to the lips and cheeks.

- You may have age spots or areas of dark pigmentation on your face. Makeup can cover these (see Chapter 14 for concealer how-tos) but will require wearing more makeup than is necessary on a daily basis. Wear sunscreen daily (also a good idea for the hands) to keep them from getting worse and keep new ones from appearing. These spots can be faded or removed; consult your dermatologist.

- Don't try to redraw your eyes with severe liner and overabundant eye shadow. Instead, use mascara and very well-blended shadows to open up the eye area. Be careful not to put too much makeup under the eye.

- Sparse brows — from decades of overplucking or from natural hormonal changes — need fill-ins of gentle color. See Chapter 14 for step-by-step instructions.

- Be careful with very matte and long-wearing lipsticks; they can be much too dry. Creamy formulas are much more flattering. For more lip definition, try a soft-colored lip pencil under your lipstick.

- Be careful with anything overly glossy or iridescent, especially on eyes and lips. However, a little gloss in the center of the lips can be very beautiful for the evening.

- Many women in their fifties have the option of continuing to color their hair to hide the gray or working with the gray. If you've decided to let your hair go gray, speak to your hair colorist about brightening it up (see Chapter 8) and be sure to alter your makeup to suit your new hair color.

Sixties and up

This stage of your life is not about making a statement with makeup, but even the lightest touch of makeup can give your face a lift and a pulled-together appearance. If you stick to the basics and blend everything well, you can't go wrong.

✔ Continue to wear sunscreen daily to prevent further age spots and skin damage. Many women opt to wear a hat for added sun protection.

✔ Recheck your foundation color often during these years. The skin tends to grow progressively paler, and you need to be sure that you still have a perfect match. Add color to your face with a creamy blusher.

✔ If you use foundation, use a small amount of a creamy, moisturizing formula that sinks into your skin rather than getting caught in the creases.

✔ Use blush and lipstick if you let your hair go gray. This is important because the absence of color in your hair can drain color from your face.

✔ Apply mascara — if you use it — with great care, because lashes can get very sparse. Instead of trying to create lashes where few exist, use mascara to give a very light coat of color and comb well.

✔ Keep your lip color soft; unless you're a lip-statement girl and always will be, avoid very dark shades, which call attention to lips that are less than perfect and make your face look paler in comparison.

Chapter 11

Finding Your Formulas and Colors

- -

In This Chapter

▶ Finding the makeup formulas that work for you

▶ Color recommendations for every type of makeup

▶ Comparing drugstore and department store makeup

▶ Visiting the makeup counter

- -

Choosing the right makeup formulas is crucial to creating your best look. If the products you use don't work with your skin type and your lifestyle, you'll never feel, or look, comfortable wearing them.

Unfortunately, deciding among makeup formulas isn't always easy. You don't have just two or three varieties of each makeup product to choose from these days; you have hundreds. This chapter explains the various formulas that are available for each makeup product and helps you find which formula will work for you. When you know what to look for and what to avoid, you save time and avoid that trial-and-error process that can be so confusing and so costly.

The element of color comes into play here, too — and so does a lot of confusion. Allow me to clear up a couple of myths: You're not a season, and there is no rule that says your makeup must match your clothes. Your makeup and clothes only need to be in harmony with one another. The key to color is to find the right shade, texture, and intensity. Repeat after me: It washes off.

Foundation

The function of foundation (also known as "base" or "makeup") is to even out your skin's tone and texture. It is *not* for masking, hiding, or recoloring your face. Foundation done right is imperceptible when it's on your skin. I've always had very sensitive skin, which isn't the best trait to have as a model.

Constantly having different types of foundation applied to my skin — and breaking out from it — made me realize how important the right formula for my skin is.

Find the right product for you based on the degree of coverage you need and the type of skin you have. The following sections break down the best formulas available (and the sidebar "Not recommended" lists a few products that I suggest you steer clear of).

Sheerest coverage

If you prefer a light, natural-looking result, try one of these formulas. If you need extra coverage on some days, you can just layer the product.

- ✔ **Water-based liquid:** Easily the most popular type of foundation. But don't be fooled — just because it's water-based doesn't mean that it doesn't contain oil; it's just made with more water than oil. Good for anyone with normal to dry skin. Blends easily to give even, natural-looking coverage. Not great for those who have oily skin, acne, or breakout problems.

- ✔ **Tinted moisturizer:** Great for everyday use — the color is just enough to even out your skin tone, and it looks like you have nothing on. Gives you three benefits in one product: evens the skin tone, moisturizes, and provides sun protection (if an SPF is included in the formulation). Blends easily and is more forgiving of less-than-perfect shade matching. Often contains oil, so women with oilier or acne-prone skin should experiment with caution. This product is great in the summer when you have a little color in your face.

- ✔ **Oil-free liquid:** Good for oily or acne-prone skin. A true oil-free formula should contain no oil whatsoever, although without an oil derivative, it may go on chalky or streaky. Many of the new high-tech foundations on the market contain silicone oils, which evaporate so completely into the skin that they're not necessarily a no-no for oily skin; look for a product that contains methicone in the ingredient listing. This foundation can be found in creamy fluid form or as a very thin, alcohol-based liquid. Works best when applied with a sponge in quick, upward strokes. It gives skin a long-lasting, matte appearance.

- ✔ **Powder-formulated foundation:** This product is great for women who want a finished but natural look and don't want to spend a lot of time getting it. Works well for normal to oily skin types.

Allergy-tested

Is your skin very dry or sensitive? Stick with allergy-tested brands of foundation; most liquids come in allergy-tested formulas. Always check the ingredient list before buying a product, and get to know which ingredients irritate your skin. You may need to experiment with several products before you find one that works well with your skin.

Most doctors recommend that women with sensitive skin stay away from these ingredients:

- Alcohol and SD alcohol
- Fragrance
- Glycols (including glycerin and propylene glycol)
- Lanolin and derivatives
- Mica
- Mineral oil and petrolatum
- Preservatives

Medium coverage

These formulas are great if you want more coverage, but they can also be blended way down on certain areas of the face to give the appearance of sheerer makeup:

- **Cream:** Brings radiance to dry or mature skins, although it may settle in lines. Can be used for full coverage or very sheer coverage. Women with oily skin should use with caution — it can make your skin appear much too shiny and can even clog pores or cause your skin to break out.

- **Oil-based liquid:** Contains more oil than water. These foundations move easily over the skin but can be a bit thick and heavy if not blended well. Great for very dry and mature skins because their extra emollience keeps in the skin's own moisture. Can give a high degree of coverage if applied generously, although it can settle in lines.

Fullest coverage

Pancake or **stick makeup** is great for applying over your regular foundation on areas that need extra coverage, such as age spots, scars, or dark pigmentation. It can also double as concealer. It's not the best choice for real life, however; it's much too heavy and only suffocates the skin. But it's great for stage and film or special effects makeup.

Not recommended

- **Long-wearing/budgeproof makeup:** Does not blend, does not look natural, and is unnecessarily harsh on the skin.

- **Wet/dry makeup:** Use this foundation dry and it looks floury on skin; use it wet and it tends to look too thick. Use the two together and you take away all the natural texture and highlight that make skin beautiful.

- **Cream-to-powder or liquid-to-powder (two-in-one formula):** This product gives you only one end result. It's better to have separate foundation and powder so that *you* have control over the final effect. If you're looking to eliminate one step, try using either foundation without powder or powder without foundation.

- **Multiphase makeup:** That stuff that settles into two distinct parts that you have to shake to mix — typically alcohol or water on top, talc and pigment on the bottom. Looks dry and chalky on the skin, but may work for acne-scarred skin.

Keep the weather in mind as you choose a foundation formula. If the sun shines year-round in your area, make sure to purchase a product with an SPF. If your area enjoys all four seasons, you may want to go a bit sheerer, or even oil-free, in the summer, and then in winter, you may want to try something a little creamier to counterbalance the air's dryness. You *must* change your formula to keep up with your skin's needs, whether seasonal or long-term (boosting emollience as skin gets older, for example). Skin changes from day to day and year to year, so be sure to give it what it needs.

Extra helps

Foundation formulas have become so specialized that you can find products that do double, even triple duty for the skin — and help you pare down steps, products, and expense. Foundation "extras" can include

- **AHAs/BHA:** Yes, they're everywhere, and foundation is no exception. Although the concentration of alpha- and beta-hydroxy acids in most foundations is nowhere near the amount found in serious skin care products, they can have a mild exfoliant effect (see Chapter 2 for more on AHAs and BHA). Be careful, though, if you're already using other AHA/BHA products: Overuse of these ingredients irritates the skin. Avoid the eye area altogether.

- **Antioxidants:** Adding these vitamins to foundations puts free-radical fighters right at the skin's surface (see Chapter 2 for an explanation of how antioxidants work). Derivatives of vitamins A, C, and E are the most commonly used antioxidant ingredients (also called retinol, ascorbic acid, and tocopherol, respectively). Women with sensitive skin may want to avoid antioxidants — breakouts may occur.

✔ **Moisturizers:** Drier skin benefits from any number of moisturizing ingredients, typically some type of oil. These emollients provide a lightweight shield that keeps your skin's natural moisture from evaporating — and your skin feeling comfortable.

✔ **Oil absorbers:** If you have very oily skin and a problem with shine reappearing throughout the day, look for ingredients like kaolin (clay) and talc. Both work to absorb excess facial oil and help the skin retain a matte appearance. However, these ingredients may also settle into fine lines.

✔ **SPF:** Many tinted moisturizers and liquid foundations come with sunscreen built right in — a great way to shield the skin from daily incidental sun exposure. You'll find, however, that some foundations contain an SPF of 8 or 10 rather than the benchmark SPF 15: That's because some sunscreen ingredients can make a product feel thick or heavy. Tinted moisturizers usually contain the highest SPFs yet still give enough coverage to even out the skin tone.

Makeup artist Glenn Marziali cautions that foundations containing titanium dioxide sunscreens can make dark skins appear ashy. For best results, look for a foundation with alternative sunscreen ingredients, or layer a foundation without an SPF over a separate sunscreen that doesn't contain the problematic ingredient.

Foundation shades

Foundation must match your natural skin tone. A color that's too light, too dark, too *anything,* is immediately noticeable, which defeats the entire purpose. You should never see foundation, only its effect — skin that looks natural, healthy, and even in tone and texture. Don't make the mistake of buying a foundation without trying it on. Trying it on allows you to see whether the foundation blends perfectly with your skin and has the texture and coverage you want.

Because most drugstores don't allow foundation testing, I recommend that you either insist on returning a color that's not perfect (even if you've used it a few times) or go to a department store or makeup boutique for this purchase. You may spend more time and money, but you can't skimp on this makeup item. Don't give up until you find the perfect shade. Your foundation is almost a part of you; if it looks wrong, nothing else that you put on your face looks right. For starters, remember these few basic rules.

For lighter skin tones:

✔ Pink-toned foundations *do not* make you look healthy, nor do they "correct" yellow tones. Pass on these.

✔ If your face is markedly lighter than your neck (which sometimes results from Retin-A and other treatment products), go one or two tones deeper with your foundation to help even out the contrast, and blend with the skin of your neck.

✔ Even if you wear sunscreen, skin tends to take on more color in summer no matter how much you avoid the sun. If you do get a bit of a tan (or if you self-tan), get a second foundation shade — or skip foundation altogether and just dot on concealer where needed.

For darker skin tones:

✔ A common problem for women with dark skin is that the skin in different areas can vary greatly in tone. Skin on the forehead and chin and around the eyes and mouth is usually the darkest, whereas the cheeks can be lighter — a situation that makes choosing a foundation color decidedly difficult. According to makeup artist Fran Cooper, "If you try to match foundation to your lighter areas, it's going to look ashy over darker spots; if you try to make everything the dark tone, it's going to look like a mask. You need a mid-tone between the two. A good way to find it is to look at the color of your neck and go with a foundation close to that shade."

Makeup artist Glenn Marziali suggests another option: Use a darker foundation on the outer areas of your face (your temples, jawline, and cheekbones) and a lighter shade in your T-zone area.

✔ Before you apply foundation, you need to "bring up" darker areas by using a concealer that's a few shades lighter, but it's fine to leave a little variation in tone. You don't want to erase your skin's natural qualities: You're just trying to achieve a more balanced overall look.

✔ If your skin is very dark, avoid foundations containing ingredients like talc or titanium dioxide, which may give your face an ashy appearance. If your skin's tone and texture are even, you may want to skip foundation altogether. Better to be your natural self than to put on a shade that looks obvious.

Custom blending

Custom-blending of foundation has become more widespread in the last few years. While this *haute couture* approach to makeup is undeniably enticing, the color-match is only as good as the salesperson who blends the product for you.

Undertones

One of the biggest buzzwords in makeup is *undertone.* All skins have one: Most common is a yellowish cast to the complexion (orange, red, blue, and green are other possibilities), and most foundation formulas are based on those shades. But try to figure out *your* undertone, and you'll likely get a different answer from everyone you ask. However, most makeup artists *do* agree that yellow works for just about everyone, and that "correcting" undertones is unnecessary for real life — that using corrective tints in shades like green and mauve is pretty tricky for the average person to pull off. So relax; undertone ambiguity is not going to make or break you. Once you find a foundation that blends flawlessly with your skin, you've done all you need to do.

Trying and buying

Your biggest single makeup expense should be your foundation. Foundation shopping is an important process, so do it at a time when you're not feeling rushed. Here's the most efficient way to get the job done:

1. **Arrive at the counter wearing no foundation and toting your own small, hand-held mirror.**

2. **After you find a formula you like, choose three or four shades that are close to your skin tone.**

3. **Swatch each color onto your face near the jawline (not your hand!) and blend.**

4. **Go outside into natural daylight and check what you've applied in your hand-held mirror.**

   Daylight is the real test for seeing whether color is a perfect match. Check your jawline. Whichever color disappears flawlessly into your skin is the winner.

   If you're really having trouble finding a shade that works for you, seek the advice of a professional (such as a makeup artist or salesperson), keeping in mind that these people are there to sell you products and probably work on commission. Take their advice with a grain of salt or go shopping with a friend who has a good eye for color.

5. **Go back to the counter, clean your skin, and then reapply the matching shade all over your face.**

   Even if you rarely wear full-face foundation in real life, do it now. See how it works with your skin for at least a half-hour before you buy.

   You may even want to try out a shade for a few days. Foundation is rarely given out as a sample — even when it is, it's probably not your shade — but if you take a small vial with you to the counter, the salesperson will usually let you take a little home.

Go through this try-on process on a fairly regular basis. You'll keep up with new innovations in formula and perhaps find an even better match. Remember, skin tone and texture change over time because of seasonal and hormonal changes, so the foundation that was right for you a year ago may not be right for you now.

Concealer

Because of its heavier, more opaque texture, concealer is the right choice for covering flaws and areas of discoloration that foundation can't hide on its own. The skin around the eyes is thinner and tends to appear darker, so most women use concealer sparingly around the eyes to look more rested and to even out the skin. If you can get away with it, skip foundation and just use concealer. Less makeup on the skin is always better.

Concealer doesn't have to be used with powder or worn with any other makeup at all. When I'm really pressed for time, whether it's day or evening, the one thing I don't leave the house without is a little concealer under my eyes and something on my lips. This way, even if I'm not made up, I look rested and pulled-together.

When choosing your concealer formula, keep in mind how you'll be wearing it, how much coverage you need, and the degree of emollience that goes with your skin type. You don't want too dry a texture, but you don't want too greasy a texture, either. Table 11-1 describes the most common types of concealer.

Table 11-1		Concealer Formulas	
Type	**Coverage**	**Positives**	**Negatives**
Liquid (tube or wand)	Sheer	Provides light, emollient coverage	Can wear off easily and collect in fine lines
Cream (pot or compact)	Sheer to medium	Gives even, lasting correction with good opacity; can be used with or without powder	Can crease and gather in lines if the formula is too heavy or greasy
Stick	Medium to full	Excellent coverage of most skin flaws and dark circles; drier formulas can be used without powder	Formulas vary widely, so you have to experiment to find one that suits you

Type	Coverage	Positives	Negatives
Corrective	Total	Complete coverage of even the most severe discoloration and scarring	Can be very heavy and difficult to blend to a natural look

You'll notice that although foundation comes in dozens of colors, concealer's shade range is much more limited. That's because you use it only to "bring up" small areas so that they blend with the rest of your face, and that doesn't require an exact color match. Because the most common flaws show up as darker tones on your skin — undereye circles, pimples, broken capillaries — a concealer that's one to two shades lighter than your foundation helps even out these areas.

A rare few women have the opposite problem, with areas (usually under the eye) that are much lighter than the rest of the face. If that description fits you, go for a concealer that's the *same* shade as your foundation or *slightly* deeper to make these areas less noticeable.

When choosing a concealer, keep in mind that yellow and neutral beige undertones are pretty foolproof for most skin tones. In the end, all that matters is whether the concealer looks natural and does the job.

 Regardless of their skin tone, some women insist on using the lightest concealer they can find. But all you really need is a concealer that's one or two shades lighter than your skin tone. Or if you don't like the thick texture of concealer and you have good skin, you can just use your foundation as a concealer.

Powder

Powder is important for giving the face a finished look. It sets foundation and concealer in place, helps other powder products glide on easier, prevents creamy products from creasing, gives skin a smooth-looking texture — and even erases makeup blunders such as too much blush. You don't *have to* use powder, but without it, makeup doesn't last as long. Powder is also great to use on bare skin to help matte down your own natural shine.

Most makeup artists use loose powder, whereas most women prefer to have pressed power, which is pressed into a compact (Table 11-2 gives the details about both types). I recommend having both: loose for your makeup at home, and pressed to carry in your purse. This way, you get the advantage of setting your makeup with a finely milled, professional-looking powder, which looks more natural, and yet you still have something in your purse for touch-ups.

> ## Portable powder
>
> Many women double up on powder, keeping loose powder at home because it's too big and messy for travel and using pressed powder for quick touch-ups throughout the day. You *can* get away with just one. To make loose powder portable, sift a little into a small plastic jar with a wide mouth and a screw-on top; apply with a brush or disposable puff (available in most drugstores). To make your pressed powder act like loose powder, swirl your powder brush around on the surface until you pick up enough, and then dust it all over your face.

Table 11-2		Powder Formulas	
Type	*Coverage*	*Positives*	*Negatives*
Loose	Sheer to full, depending on application	Very light; easy to apply and blend; widest shade selection	Can wear off easily; looks cakey if not blended well
Pressed	Sheer to full, depending on application	Very portable; ideal for fast touch-ups	Usually contains some type of oil, so oily skin should look for powders that are specially formulated for oily skin; can look chalky if not blended well

Powders with iridescence or sparkle shouldn't be used all over the face. They're wonderful for highlighting cheekbones, bustline, and shoulders, however, especially in the evening. Older women need to be careful with this product, which tends to settle in lines.

Like foundation, powder must be tried on if you're going to find your best color match. (Yep, it's another investment, but well worth it.) Because powder comes in such an assortment of shades, not to mention undertones and textures, trying on really is the only way to be sure that it looks right on your skin.

The choices can be confusing. You'll find dozens of powders in realistic skin-toned shades (pretty self-explanatory). You'll find translucent powders that come in just a few colors. You'll also find powders with obvious undertones of yellow, pink, peach, and even green. As with foundation, you really don't need to get into these "corrective" shades — just find a powder that matches your natural skin tone, follow these basic rules, and you're all set:

Translucent powder

"Translucent" does not equal "transparent," so these powders are *not* invisible on the skin. Although translucent powders contain *less* pigment than regular powder products (making them more forgiving if you haven't chosen your perfect powder shade), they do contain a certain degree of color, so they must be tried on before purchasing. Selection is usually limited to "light," "medium," and "dark," so you may not be able to find an exact match, especially if you have very dark skin.

✔ Don't try to recolor your complexion with powder. A too-light shade doesn't give you a "flawless" look; it gives you a floury finish. And a powder that's too dark doesn't take the edge off a pale complexion — it just makes you look like you need to wash your face.

✔ If your skin is very oily or very dry, you must use a powder that works with your skin type to get the most natural, lasting effect. Breakout shine can be held at bay with added oil-control ingredients; extra moisturizers make a big difference in how powder looks and feels on dry skin.

Before you try on a powder, you need to keep in mind *how* you'll be using it. If you usually wear powder on bare skin, try your powder the same way. If you wear foundation on a regular basis, you should try on the powder *over* foundation so that you can see the final color and effect.

Follow these steps to find the perfect powder shade:

1. **Arrive at the counter wearing your regular foundation and no powder (or with bare skin if you're not a foundation-wearer), and with your trusty hand-held mirror.**

2. **Find a powder formula that's compatible with your skin type.**

3. **Choose a few shades that are close to your natural skin tone.**

4. **Apply each shade to a different area of the face (say, one on your forehead and another on your right cheek).**

5. **Step out into natural daylight to see the results.**

   Not only are you looking for color, but you're also looking for texture: Reject any powder that's heavy, chalky, shiny, or doesn't blend in to look like real skin. When you find a powder that looks and feels completely natural, that's the one you want.

6. **If possible, wear the powder for a while before you buy it to make sure that its texture, color, and shine control properties remain constant.**

Powder blotting papers (available at specialty drugstores) are wonderful. Used professionally to keep the skin shine-free without overusing powder, they're economical and small enough to fit in the tiniest purses.

Blush

Blush has two basic functions: to add a healthy-looking glow to the face, and to give subtle enhancement to the cheekbones. The best blush looks totally natural once it's on, so choose a product with a texture that blends perfectly into your skin. Table 11-3 gives you your options.

Table 11-3		**Blush Formulas**	
Type	*Texture*	*Positives*	*Negatives*
Powder	Dry; applied with a brush	Easiest to control and blend; widest color selection; great for almost every type of skin	Can look chalky on very dry skin
Cream	Creamy; applied with fingers or a sponge	Gives radiant, natural-looking color; blends easily; especially good for dry and mature skin	Color will not last on oily skin
Gel/Liquid	Wet; applied with fingers	Long-lasting color; good for oily skin	Tricky to apply; must moisturize before applying and blend quickly to avoid streaking; can stain skin

Blush has always been my favorite makeup. I love to use cream blush with powder blush on top, or mix up the colors to create my own. It's a great way to keep your makeup fresh and change it a bit from season to season. If you don't have different colors of blush or cream blusher, try using lipsticks alone or blended down under your powder blush to change the color.

The best blush seems to be a natural part of your skin — and as luck would have it, nature has provided a couple nifty tricks for finding that magical shade. The easiest is to take a look at your cheeks right after you've exercised. Your natural lip color is also a good indicator of your best blush shade. For most women with light-to-medium skin tones, the most realistic-looking blush colors are pink, rose, apricot, and peach. Trying it on, as always, is the best indicator: You may even find a couple shades (one more pink, one more tawny) that work for you. Even lavenders mixed with pinks can create beautiful shades.

If your skin is very dark, your face may not show an obvious flushed cheek to go by, but that doesn't mean that you can't wear blush. Look for richly pigmented shades like wine or plum, or even brown tones like bronze or umber, to give your cheeks a bit of added glow. Try on the blush to make sure that it doesn't leave an ashy or shiny look on your skin.

A few more helpful blush-color hints:

- ✔ **Don't limit yourself to just one blush.** If you have a favorite shade, try it in different textures — powder, cream — to create different effects. And don't be afraid to try different tones of blush: Apricot and pink may look equally good on you, and having a choice provides a great way to vary your look for different moods or seasons.

- ✔ **Bronzer can be blush's best friend.** You can use bronzer (see Chapter 14) to tawny-up your usual blush shade when you're tan, or mix a little with a too-loud shade to tone it down.

- ✔ **Avoid blush that contains obvious sparkle.** If you want to enhance your cheekbones with a little shimmer, it's always better to add a little powder or stick highlighter after your blush is on. See Chapter 14 for application tips.

Eyebrow Makeup

If your brows constantly need major fill-ins, it's worth getting a product created specifically for the task. A good eyebrow pencil has a drier, more matte texture than an eyeliner pencil (which, after all, is made for smudging) and is good for creating the look of individual hairs. Powder brow color is better than powder eye shadow for creating an illusion of thickness. It has a rich, matte texture and comes in shades that match natural brow hair and stay true once blended.

Brow grooming

Clear brow gel is a hot product these days, but you can always use a little hairspray or hair gel in place of it. Put the hairspray or hair gel directly on an eyebrow brush and then, while it's still wet, brush brows into place.

Brow gels are a wonderful addition to brow grooming and styling. Most are applied with a mascara-style wand with or without fill-in underneath, and are great for helping brows look thicker and well-groomed. Check out Table 11-4 to find what *you* need.

Table 11-4		Brow Color Formulas	
Type	*Texture*	*Positives*	*Negatives*
Pencil	Creamy; applied right from the pencil	Good for creating the look of brow hairs where none exist; perfect for redrawing the brow	Not as lasting as powder color unless set with loose powder
Powder	Dry; applied with an angle brush	Blends well with existing brow hair; easy to apply; wide selection of colors; long-lasting	Not right for re-creating absent brows
Gel	Moist, gel form applied with a wand	Helps brows look thicker and stay in place	Doesn't look nice on very sparse brows; can look stiff if overused

Remember, texture is important here. Don't use any product that looks shiny, feels greasy, or leaves a strange undertone on the skin after it's applied.

For natural-looking brows, most women should choose a shade of pencil or powder that's slightly lighter than their own brow hair. Matching your hair shade exactly is usually impossible, anyway — and going darker only gives a harsh, drawn-on effect (the same holds true even if you have black brows — use a deep brown for fill-ins instead).

However, there are a few exceptions to the rule. If your brows are blonde to the point of extinction, use a very light brown or taupe shade to strengthen them. And if your brow hairs are white, adding more white would look very strange indeed. Instead, use a light shade of gray.

Eye Shadow

Although you have a few varieties of eye shadows to choose from (see Table 11-5), powder shadow is the overwhelming favorite for its ease of application. It's also the only shadow product that you can place precisely for shading and shaping the eye. Most women choose eye shadow on the basis of color only, but you need to keep three other factors in mind:

- ✔ **Texture:** Eye shadow should be smooth and silky and blend easily over the skin. Avoid anything that feels dry, scratchy, or grainy.

- ✔ **Finish:** Finish simply refers to whether the product is matte or contains shine. Matte is a classic and is best for everyday wear; a little shimmer is nice for summer, evening, or simply for a change.

  Women with sensitive or mature eyes or contact lenses may want to avoid shimmery shadows. They usually contain mica, a finely ground mineral that can flake into eyes and cause redness and irritation.

- ✔ **Intensity:** Comes from the amount of pigment put into the formula: The more pigment, the denser the color. Anyone who's ever tried to create a dramatic, smoky, black eye is familiar with this phenomenon: You put on layer after layer of color, but the effect is never as deep or rich as you want. That's because there's not enough *black* in your black — there's too little pigment and too much filler.

Table 11-5		Eye Shadow Formulas	
Type	*Texture*	*Positives*	*Negatives*
Powder	Dry; applied with an eye shadow brush	Easy to place and blend; limitless colors; the best choice for sculpting the eye with color; can be used wet or dry	Can look obvious if not well-blended; may fall underneath the eye when being applied
Cream (pot, wand, tube)	Smooth and moist; usually applied with a finger	Gives a very soft look; quick and easy to use	Not good for precise color placement; can collect in creases
Shadow pencil	Creamy and smudgy; thicker and more emollient than pencil eyeliner	Very portable; gives a smudgier effect than powder or cream	Not very lasting due to higher oil content; can crease and smear easily

Literally thousands of eye shadow shades are available, but for basic eye-enhancing purposes, think in terms of *three.* To properly shape the eye, you need complementary shadow colors in three different intensities:

- ✔ A dark shade to define the crease (which can also be used for lining)

- ✔ A medium shade to use all over the lid

- ✔ A light shade to highlight smaller areas of the eye

These three shades must blend together easily, so stay within the same basic color family. You'll never go wrong if you stick to neutral hues: Earth tones like black, gray, navy, and brown are the basis for most neutral shadow shades and can be found in a wide range of tones and intensities. Considered "The Classics," they all work together and look great on everyone.

A few other guidelines that everyone can use:

✔ **Remember that your natural skin tone has an impact on how shadow looks.** Color shows up more intensely on very light skin, so be careful with deep hues. Very dark skin, however, needs rich, saturated shades in order for color to show up on the lid.

✔ **A shadow shade that matches your skin tone is always good to have on hand.** When you want a fast, finished-looking eye, one quick sweep of color is all you need.

✔ **Matching your eye shadow to your iris does not make your eye color stand out.** You must create a *contrast* for your eye color to look more pronounced.

✔ **Those kits with 1,001 eye shadows that you get as a gift with purchase or for a small additional cost are a great way to find colors that you may never think to buy.** Those colors may end up working for you.

✔ **If you want to use a bit of shimmer, keep it subtle.** Remember that shinier textures highlight imperfections. Mature women should be cautious with this effect.

✔ **Colorful shades — like blue, green, purple — *can* look great if you keep it simple.** Stick to one shade, blend it to the sheerest suggestion of color, and use related neutral tones if you need to deepen or highlight other areas of the lid.

Eyeliner

The Egyptians knew the power of a good eyeliner, though their formula — charcoal, tree resins, and ground beetles — probably wasn't so great for their eyes. Liner is unbeatable for shaping and balancing the look of the eyes and for making the lashes appear thicker.

With eyeliner, the main thing to consider is the effect you want to achieve. Do you want soft, smudgy definition or a very sharp, intense line? Pencil or shadow used wet or dry gives the softest effect, while cake or liquid liner gives a stronger, more intense effect. Table 11-6 discusses the pros and cons of the various types.

Lining the inside rim of the eye

Marlene Dietrich did it. Brigitte Bardot did it. And I do it. Your ophthalmologist may not be pleased, but the time has come to discuss lining the inside rim of the eye.

Using liner inside the eye can enhance the look of many different types of eye makeup, but it can also lead to irritation or infection. Always keep your eye pencils clean and well sharpened — but not dangerously pointy — for sterilization.

Four colors work best for this purpose:

✔ **Black** gives a sexy, smoky look that's best when the rest of your eye makeup is intense. (Be careful: It also makes small eyes look smaller.)

✔ **Brown** is a toned-down, softer version of black.

✔ **White** can help brighten and "open" the eye by visually extending the white area. Use it when you want to appear wide-eyed. This effect looks best in low light.

✔ **Beige** also creates the illusion of a larger white area to the eye, and it gives a more subtle effect than white liner.

Table 11-6	Eyeliner Formulas		
Type	*Texture*	*Positives*	*Negatives*
Shadow	Dry; applied wet or dry with a brush or sponge-tip applicator	Very versatile; used dry, gives softest definition; used wet, gives stronger, more lasting color	Hard to build up intensity unless the pigment is very strong
Pencil	Creamy; strokes on right from the pencil	Applies and blends easily; creates effects from subtle to strong; available in smudge-proof formulas	Smudges and fades into the skin; dry pencils pull the skin around the eye
Cake/ liquid/pen	Goes on wet; applied with a small brush	Creates a bold, intense line; long-lasting	Tricky to apply; can look harsh

Whatever your skin tone or hair color, eyeliner in classic, neutral colors is always the best choice. Shades of black, gray, brown, and navy really do work for just about everyone and are foolproof favorites for everyday wear. Dozens of shades are available within this color range, so try a few and see how you like their different effects: Blondes often prefer a brown liner for day and black for more impact at night, while many women with gray hair like the way charcoal gray complements their coloring. You'll find that most shades come in matte textures; leave the sparkle and iridescence for eye shadows.

If you'd like to use a more colorful liner — a moss green, perhaps, or a dusky eggplant tone — keep the shade deep, subtle, and well-blended.

Mascara

Thick, dark lashes are considered a sign of sensuality and youth. Mascara is basically a mixture of pigments, waxes, and oils; the best-loved types come in gel and creamy consistencies and a basic range of colors. When buying mascara, the real questions are "What do you need it to do?" and "How long do you want it to stay on?"

- ✔ **Lengthening** mascara's main concern is making the lashes look longer. Stay away from brands that contain rayon or nylon fibers.

- ✔ **Thickening** formulas tend to be a bit heavier because they build up a volumizing coat of color on lashes. Clumping can be a problem with these mascaras, so always comb well after applying.

- ✔ **Conditioning** formulas contain added ingredients that are supposed to improve lash health. Remember, lashes are like any other hair — no matter how many proteins or vitamins you apply on the outside, they won't grow thicker, faster, or longer. However, if you like how these formulas make your lashes feel, then they certainly can't hurt.

Table 11-7	Mascara Formulas		
Type	**Point of Difference**	**Positives**	**Negatives**
Water-soluble	Comes off in water	Good staying power; wide variety of choices and effects; best choice for daily wear	Runs if exposed to tears, sweat, or rain
Waterproof	Won't come off in water	Stays on through swimming and tears	Contains ingredients that can dry and break the lashes; must be removed with a special solvent
Cake	Dry, pressed powder; add water and then apply with a small brush	Gives a very thick look to the lashes	Tricky to apply; can look too matte and unnatural
Lash darkener/ Clear mascara	Contains little or no pigment	Very natural, glossy look; great for young girls	Doesn't thicken or lengthen; not great for pale or faded lashes

No earth-shattering news about color here: Black and brown mascara work for just about everyone. If your lashes are naturally dark, black will see you through just about anything. Brown is a nice option if you want to give the eyes a softer look, and it's usually a better color match for blondes and redheads. You may also want to try a clear mascara when you want to enhance the gloss of your lashes without adding color.

Lip Color

You'll find a zillion different lip colors, but they all pretty much come down to the same three ingredients: waxes, oils, and dyes. In general, the higher a product's oil content, the glossier the finish. Lip gloss contains so much oil that it can't be molded into solid form, whereas the new long-wearing lipsticks contain so little oil that you may need a little lip balm underneath to get them to go on smoothly. Between those two extremes are an infinite variety of options; Table 11-8 narrows it down to the most common types. Base your choice on the look and staying power that appeal to you.

Table 11-8			Lip Color Formulas	
Type	*Coverage*	*Finish*	*Positives*	*Negatives*
Gloss/ Gloss stick	Very sheer	Shiny	Goes on quickly and easily; application doesn't have to be precise	Wears off quickly; hard to keep in place; can bleed into fine lines
Sheer	Natural	Moist	Gives lips a light, fresh-looking stain of color	Doesn't give very lasting or full coverage
Cream	Medium to full	Smooth	Comfortable and easy to wear; widest selection of colors; can be used to create many different effects	Not the longest-lasting option
Matte	Full	Matte	Very lasting, intense color	Can be dry and difficult to apply
Long-wearing	Opaque	Very matte	Very long-lasting color and ultra-matte finish	Can be very drying; color may peel away from lips
Pencil (liner)	Medium to full	Matte	Long lasting; can be used to color lips on its own, or to help keep other lip color in place; best tool for correcting lip shape	Can give lips a dry look and feel if applied all over

Lip fix-its

If lipstick migration is a real problem for you, a multitude of lipstick-fix products are made to keep color in place: Some are used as a base *under* lipstick; others go over lipstick as a final "sealing" coat. However, you may not need to buy these specialized products to keep your lipstick in line. Makeup artist Glenn Marziali suggests applying a little concealer with powder or smoothing on some lip balm before applying lipstick to keep the color from wandering.

Even if you have one favorite *color* you come back to time and again, have fun experimenting with different textures and finishes. Sheer stains are great in the summer or for a more natural look; matte textures give a very polished effect; a quick slick of gloss makes any pair of lips look fresh. And you should always have at least one neutral, lip-toned pencil on hand for shaping and keeping your other color products in place.

Many lip color products now have built-in SPFs — a bonus that's really worth taking advantage of. Because the lips have little protective *melanin* (the stuff that makes skin tan), they're a prime site for skin cancer — and sunlight is also one of the main triggers for cold sores. These all-in-one formulas are worth taking advantage of, especially if you're snow-skiing or are in constant sun exposure.

Your best lip color? Any shade that makes you feel pretty and gives you confidence. I know that sounds a bit simplistic, but because makeup's whole purpose is to help you feel good about your looks, I'm not going to steal your bright orange lipstick if it *really* makes you happy. (I will, however, say that natural tones are much more flattering.) Here are a few simple guidelines to help you make sense of all the color options out there:

✔ **Everyone needs a good, everyday lip color that always looks right.** To find it, look at the color of your bare lips, and then try lipstick in a similar shade while wearing little other makeup on your face. Any shade that looks like a natural part of you is a keeper.

✔ **Everyone needs at least one lip pencil.** You may, in fact, need a few. The basic is in a neutral shade close to your natural lip color; you'll use it when you want to give your lips a subtle reshape and to keep lip color in line. If you wear very bright or dark shades of lipstick, matching pencils give you the most perfect edge.

- **The only way to see whether a color is good for you is to try it on.** Getting a basic color impression by slicking color onto the back of your hand is fine, but after you find a favorite, try it on. The color will look different on your lips and against your face, so trying is a must.

- **In general, the deeper your skin tone, the deeper your lipstick shade should be.** Very light skins should stick to the gentler end of the spectrum, while darker tones need to go for more intensity in order for color to be seen.

- **If you like a certain color, try it in different textures.** Using your beloved pink as a matte, a cream, a shimmer, or a gloss adds variety to your look.

- **Don't worry about matching your lip color to your blush.** Just keep them in the same basic color family.

- **If you like dark colors but feel like they're too much every time you put them on, try just staining your lips with them.** Apply the color (don't worry if it's much darker than you'd like), wait five minutes, and then blot it down. It should leave a lighter version of what you put on. Use lip balm on top for moisture.

- **Learn to understand your mouth and which colors enhance your lips, skin tone, and hair.** The thinner your lips, the more neutral your lipstick color should be.

- **Mixing colors is the best way to vary your lip shade and fine-tune the color until it's perfect.**

Red alert

Ever the classic, red lipstick is in a category all its own — so of course it has its own rules:

- Wearing red lipstick is all about finding the right shade. You'll find true blue-reds, orange-reds, even reds with brown undertones. Don't get discouraged if you haven't found the right one. You may have to try several variations, but you *will* find one for you.

- Not all red mouths have to be a deep, saturated matte red. You can mix a red pencil and sheer gloss for a less serious, shiny red, or blot down a creamy red 'til it leaves just a hint of color on your lips.

- Deeply pigmented shades of red can stain the lips, especially if you wear these reds on a daily basis. A base of foundation or a lip-fix product can help prevent the problem, as can scrupulous removal of all color at night. (See Chapter 15 for more tips for stained lips.)

- Avoid true-red shades if your face is blotchy, irritated, or ruddy — your lips will only draw attention to the redness in your skin.

- With red lipstick, liner makes it easier to create the perfect shape. Use a pencil shade that matches your lipstick, or a neutral, to create the desired shape.

Organizing your lipsticks

Rather than having 20 tubes of lipstick in your drawer that you never use, dig out or cut off a chunk of color with a toothpick and smoosh it into a small, compartmentalized container (find them at beauty supply stores, drugstores, and even hardware stores). This is a great way to not only organize what you have but also create new colors by mixing shades together. It also lets you use up the last bits of colors you love, and it's great for travel, too.

Shopping for Your Makeup

You can find great makeup in many different places. All the following resources should be available to you unless you reside in a very remote location; then you'll need to take advantage of other shopping resources (see Appendix B for contact information for hundreds of companies).

- **Drugstores** carry a selection of makeup, but that selection usually depends on the size of the store.

- **Department stores** usually carry many different brands in a range of prices.

- **Beauty boutiques** are stores dedicated to one particular brand.

- **Beauty salons** sometimes offer makeup as an adjunct to hair care and other products.

- **Beauty supply stores** stock specialty and professional items for cosmetologists, but they usually let non-pros shop, too.

- **Direct sales** includes television, catalog, over-the-phone ordering, and door-to-door.

Drugstore versus department store

Easily the two most accessible and popular makeup sources for women, drugstores and department stores differ in three main ways: service, product testing, and price.

- **Drugstores** are typically self-service with no sales assistance, they rarely have tester units available, and products are usually inexpensive.

- **Department stores** have at-counter help, testers for most products, and prices that range from reasonable to stratospheric.

Now for the big question: Does it matter where you buy your makeup? Yes and no — but only for certain types of products, or if you need a service that only a department store or makeup boutique can provide.

Go to the department store or makeup boutique for . . .

- **Foundation and powder:** These two items (your biggest makeup expenditures) should always be tested on the face — and some drugstores don't allow try-ons.

- **Service and support:** If you're the type of person who likes to ask a lot of questions or get one-on-one help, you can find it here. Super-shopper trick: Take down a makeup counter's phone number and call when you need to restock on favorites — they'll ship products right to your door and save you a trip.

- **Sampling products:** You can play to your heart's content among the testers. Just use caution: Product testers can harbor germs, so never use them in the eye or lip areas, which are very prone to infection.

- **Nice-looking packaging:** That's what a lot of the money you spend here actually goes for, as well as to marketing and advertising costs.

Go to the drugstore for . . .

- **Mascara:** It's cheaper, and drugstores have a huge selection. Because you have to throw the stuff out every few months, why break the bank? (However, if you have sensitive eyes, you may want to stick with department stores in case you need to return a mascara that you find unusable.)

- **Basic makeup helpers:** The little extras that get you through application: cotton swabs, cotton pads, latex sponges, facial tissues, and pencil sharpeners.

- **A cheap color fix:** If you've been dying to experiment with different shades for your eyes, cheeks, or lips, buy them here. You'll find many products in a variety of shades and textures.

Go where you want for the rest

Although I always prefer trying on to taking my chances, sometimes overspending just doesn't make sense. If you're using a no-brainer color — black eyeliner, after all, is black eyeliner — or you feel confident in your shade-picking prowess, by all means go nuts at the drugstore. You can make even the cheapest makeup look great if you apply it well with the proper tools.

Pencil it in

Ready for a deep, dark secret? Most eye and lip pencils are made at the same three cosmetic factories. So whether you pay 99¢ in a drugstore or $25 in a department store, you're getting basically the same product — just in different packaging. However, you still need to make sure that the shades and textures are right. Here's what to look for:

✔ Eye pencils should glide on smoothly without catching or pulling skin, but they should not be so soft that they leave a thick deposit of color, nor so greasy that the color smears and travels after the skin warms it.

✔ Eyebrow pencils should have a firm, slightly dry texture that enables them to be sharpened to a fine point.

✔ Lip-lining pencils should be soft but slightly dry. A too-greasy pencil will not hold lipstick in place, and it can feather into fine lip-area lines.

However, department store brands do tend to be more current, incorporating newer technology and eliminating annoyances like sparkle and garishness that are still evident in drugstore brands. Product textures often feel smoother, packaging is usually sturdier, and you can pretty much return products without complaint. I recommend that you compare product offerings from both places for yourself and take it from there.

No matter where you purchase makeup products, ask about the store's return policy before you buy. If they don't accept returns on makeup, consider shopping elsewhere.

Shopping tipsheet

Even after all these years of modeling, makeup shopping can make me feel like I did when I was 14: shy and unsure and afraid to upset someone. When someone says, "That looks great on you; you should really get it," it's so easy to get wrapped up in that, and to feel that you have to buy it or you're going to hurt that person's feelings. But you have to stop and listen to your own instincts. If you know how you look best, you'll be able to avoid bad advice and bad products. These tips should make the whole shopping experience easier:

✔ Make a list of what you need ahead of time.

✔ Don't wear the makeup item you're setting out to buy. Although testing a product on your hand is okay if you're only checking for texture, blendability, and general color, you want to be able to try it on your face if you find a contender.

✔ If possible, avoid shopping on weekends or at lunch times: That's when makeup-counter traffic is at its peak. Crowds slow down the whole try-and-buy process, inhibiting your access to testers and sales assistance.

✔ Not every counter has proper cleanup stuff set out, so carry a pack of travel tissues or baby wipes when you're makeup shopping.

✔ Take along a small pad and pen so that you can write down the names of products and shades that you liked but didn't buy.

✔ Check out lots of different brands, and then buy the best makeup items for your needs. Resist a salesperson who tries to sell you the entire line of *anything*. He or she is concerned about making a sale and racking up a commission — not about whether a product from another line may be better for you.

✔ Remember that cosmetic companies aren't always right. A company may make one product you love, but that doesn't mean that everything the company makes is a good choice for you.

✔ If you're not finding the answers or products that you need from a particular store or counter, look elsewhere. Don't settle for anything that is not totally comfortable and right.

Remember your tester awareness

Although the chances of catching something from a tainted tester are pretty slim, most cosmetic companies are very diligent about tester cleanliness and train their salespeople in hygienic procedures. However, that doesn't mean that your fellow shoppers always follow the rules. Before you allow something to touch your face, take a good look at the tester and the entire counter: Does it look clean and organized? Are products wiped of smudges and drips? Are disposable sampling tools — cotton balls and swabs, tissues, and makeup wedges — plentiful and easily available? These are all good signs that proper precautions are being taken.

Most companies follow these testing guidelines. You should, too — to protect yourself and the next customer.

✔ **Liquid and creamy foundations** should be dipped from the jar with a cotton swab. Don't double-dip; if you need more, use the other end or a new swab.

✔ **Compact foundations and creamy blushers** can be sampled with a disposable latex sponge, or you can use a cotton swab to transfer the product to your fingers.

✔ **Loose and pressed powders and powder blushers** can be swiped with a cotton ball and applied to the face.

✔ **Powder eye shadow** can be tested on your hand with a cotton swab.

Insider information

Staying sane while makeup shopping is much easier when you know how things work on the *other* side of the counter:

✔ Because major stores earn major profits, cosmetic companies invest more in their bigger counters — which includes hiring salespeople to work for their line *only*. (The big tip-off is a counter where all salespeople are wearing the same uniform.) Permanent sales staff receive in-depth product training and regular refresher courses — so they're usually quite knowledgeable about the products they're selling.

✔ Smaller stores usually have "floaters" who go from counter to counter. Although it's nice that they can take you through all the different brands in the store, they know a little about everything but don't have in-depth knowledge of any one line.

✔ Salespeople are trained to maximize sales — and their commission — with add-on products. They'll tell you that product A really works best when combined with products B and C. Don't fall for it. If a product doesn't work well on its own, why would you want it?

✔ **Eye and lip pencils** should be sharpened with a clean sharpener before being used on the hand; doing so removes any possible contamination from the exposed end.

✔ **Mascara** should never be offered for testing at a makeup counter; the chance for spreading infection is too high. Some companies do stock one-use disposable wands or tiny tubes for individual sampling; as long as it's for your eyes only, it's fine.

✔ **Lipstick** can be swatched onto the back of the hand for basic color-choosing; actual testing on the lips is not recommended.

Getting Out of a Rut

The dreaded Makeup Rut is a sneaky little problem that happens for many different reasons, but the result is always the same: You look frozen in time. Don't let yourself get so busy, so bored, so locked in one look that you keep yourself from trying new things. Knowing your face is one thing; doing your makeup the exact same way for 20 years is another.

You're in a rut if . . .

- ✔ You have two looks: No Makeup and Makeup, which you apply the same way every day, regardless of season or occasion.
- ✔ You can't remember the last time you bought a new makeup product.
- ✔ You can't remember the last time you bought a different makeup shade.
- ✔ You can't remember when you bought the makeup products that you're currently using (see "Nothing lasts forever," later in this chapter).
- ✔ You apply your makeup the same way you did in high school.
- ✔ You have a problem with your favorite products being discontinued.
- ✔ You find applying makeup to be a chore; it's something you *have to* do.

To get out of a rut . . .

- ✔ Go to the drugstore, buy some inexpensive new shades that you're attracted to, and play.
- ✔ Let a friend who is good with her makeup experiment on you.
- ✔ Look through beauty and fashion magazines for makeup ideas and then spend some time (a lazy Saturday afternoon is great for this) trying to re-create your favorite looks. You'll be inspired to find new ways to use your makeup.
- ✔ Have a cosmetics-counter makeover. If you love it, great. If you hate it, at least you'll know what *not* to do.
- ✔ Subtract one of your regular products from your makeup routine. Every few days, choose a different one to eliminate.
- ✔ Substitute a new product for an old standby: brown instead of black mascara; cream blush instead of powder.

Finally, rut or no rut, whether you're a lipstick-lover or a foundation-phobe, you must remember the Makeup Mantra: It washes off.

Nothing lasts forever

Even beer has an expiration date these days, but somehow makeup is considered immortal. However, products *do* go bad after a certain period of time: Dust, air, and even the bacteria from your own fingers work to deteriorate products over months of use. Using a product that's past its prime can give you everything from bad application to a bad infection, so pay attention to what you're putting on your face.

What you're looking for: anything that has an odd odor, strange discoloration, or visible mold; liquid products that have separated (unless that's how they're meant to be); or any noticeable changes in texture or consistency. In general, the more fluid the product, the shorter the shelf life, so resist the urge to stockpile liquid or cream products — they'll go bad before you can use them. You can help prolong your makeup's useful life by keeping products tightly covered and storing them in a cool, dry place. Remember: The sun is your makeup's worst enemy.

Product	Useful Life Once Opened	Prolong Life by Doing This
Fluid foundation	1 year	Store in the refrigerator or another cool place
Pressed and loose powder, powder blush, eye shadow	2 years	Store in a dry place
Mascara and liquid eyeliner	3 to 6 months	Keep tightly capped; never thin product with saliva
Lip, eye, and brow pencils	2 to 3 years	Keep covered with the cap to prevent dry-out or store in the refrigerator to keep fresh and firm
Lipstick	2 years	Store in a cool, dry place

The Makeup
Workbook

Makeup looks designed and photographed by François Nars

Makeup can seem confusing sometimes, but it's really very simple if you remember that there are three basic ways to do it: You can emphasize your eyes, you can emphasize your lips, or you can keep everything natural and in balance. Just think of Brigitte Bardot's black eyeliner, or Marilyn Monroe's red lips,

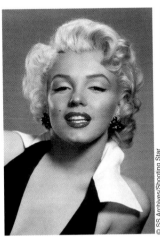
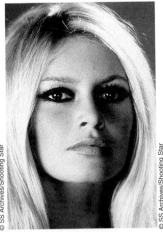
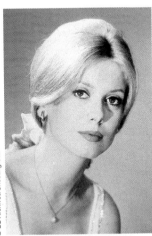
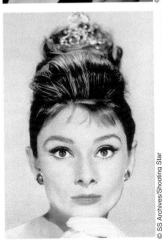
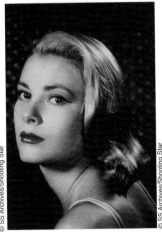
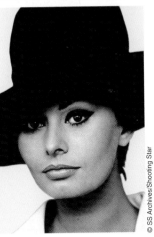

or Grace Kelly's refined makeup — they're all classic looks that have never gone out of style. For me, and many makeup artists, beauty icons from old movies or books are the greatest inspirations for creating new looks. These are just a few examples among the many icons of beauty who have inspired me. I hope that they inspire you.

natural glamour

In my everyday life, either I wear no makeup at all or I keep it very natural: usually a little mascara to brighten my eyes, concealer and blush if I need it, and lip gloss. The makeup I have on here is one of my favorite looks — it's simple, classic, and anyone can do it.

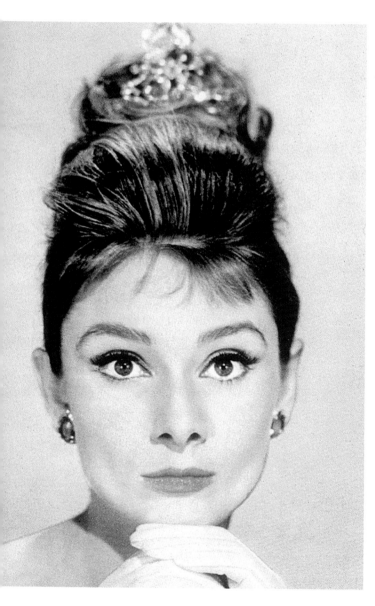

This is kind of a modernized version of the classic *Breakfast at Tiffany's* look (see Audrey Hepburn at left), but because there's no heavy liner or false lashes, it's more natural. It's just beautiful makeup that's very easy to apply (actually, I did a lot of steps myself for this photo). And if you want to take it a step further for evening, all you have to do is vary your lipstick — maybe use red, or amethyst, or peach — to change your look.

Modern *Breakfast at Tiffany's* Makeup

1. After applying a little concealer under my eyes, I used a medium-brown pencil to fill in my eyebrows and then blended it with an angle brush.

2. Next, I curled my eyelashes. My lashes tend to droop near the outer corner, so I use a corner curler to get the lift right where I need it.

3. Pale beige eye shadow was applied all over my lid to even out the color, and then a medium brown shadow was used in the crease and blended outward to give my eyes more definition.

4. Next, black eye pencil was applied all along my lash line, with the line getting slightly thicker toward the outer edge. An angle brush was used to blend and "wing" it out at the outer corner.

5. I put on two coats of black mascara, top lashes only.

6. After using a little loose powder, a natural pink blush was applied to my cheeks and blended until it disappeared into my skin.

7. I lined my lips with a neutral pink pencil, but I applied it with a lip brush so that I'd still get the emphasis, but no hard line. Over that, I put on a little beigy-pink lip gloss. Done!

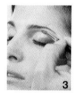

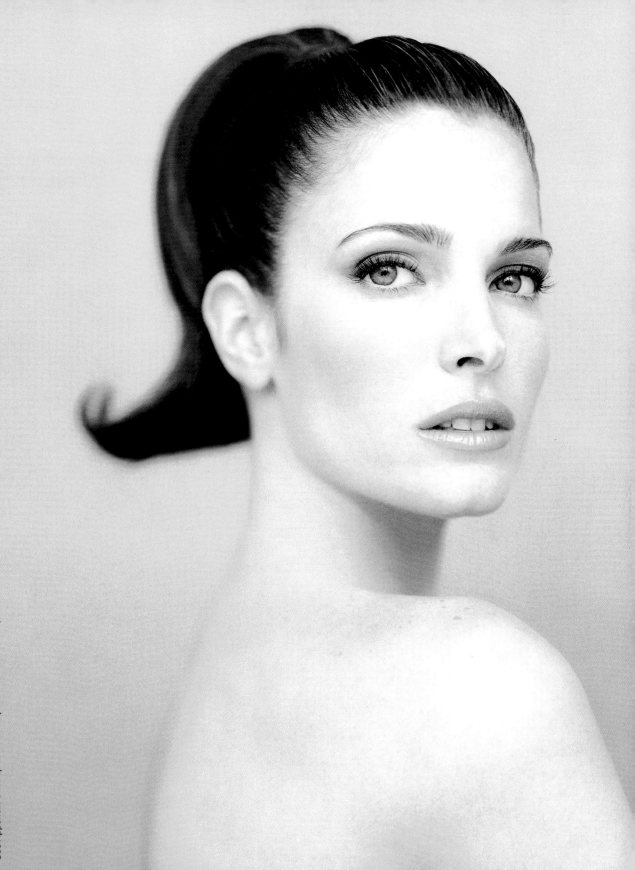

night & day

I've always thought that my mother took impeccable care of her skin, and as you can see from these pictures, all the hard work paid off. During the day, she needs very little makeup — just enough to enhance. Going from day to evening is so simple — intensifying eye makeup and defining the lip are all you really need to do.

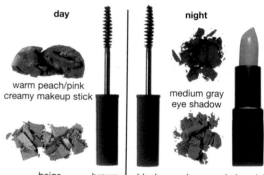

day

warm peach/pink creamy makeup stick

beige eye shadow

brown mascara

night

black mascara

medium gray eye shadow

mahogany eye shadow

beigy pink lipstick

This is a pretty, no-makeup look that's just enough for daytime, and great at any age.

Natural Day Makeup

1. After applying eye cream, tinted moisturizer was used to even out skin tone. Concealer was dotted under the eye.

2. A creamy makeup stick in a warm peach/pink shade was blended onto the apples of the cheeks.

3. Applied with a brow color brush, mahogany eye shadow was used to fill in the brows where needed.

4. Beige eye shadow was applied wet with a shadow brush and then buffed down once dry; this trick, great for mature lids, helps shadow adhere better. Next, a lighter shade of beige was applied to the inner half of the lid.

5. Lashes were curled, and then top and bottom lashes were given a coat of brown mascara.

6. Loose powder was used on the nose and chin to matte down shine.

7. The same creamy makeup stick that was used as blusher was applied to lips with a lip brush.

3

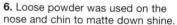

4

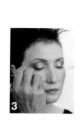

7

Here's proof that nighttime makeup doesn't have to be complicated or completely redone. The day look is simply added to, with deeper color on eyes and a touch of gloss on lips.

From Day to Evening

1. Medium gray shadow was used wet to line the eyes and then blended with an eye shadow brush once dry. The same shadow was applied dry to the outer third of the lid.

2. A little mahogany shadow was blended into the crease, winging slightly outward and upward.

3. Four clusters of false lashes were applied to the outer third of the upper lid to add a bit of drama.

4. Black mascara was applied to help blend false and natural lashes.

5. A peachy powder blush was added to give more definition to the cheekbones.

6. The face was finished with a little loose powder applied with a brush.

7. Beigy pink lipstick was applied with a brush; then a neutral lip pencil was used around the edges for definition. Lip gloss in a similar shade was used in the center of the lip for sheen.

3

4

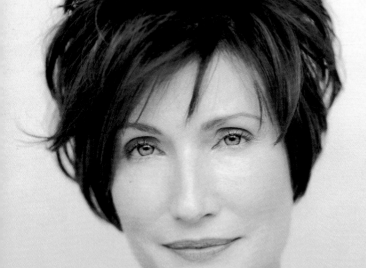

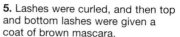

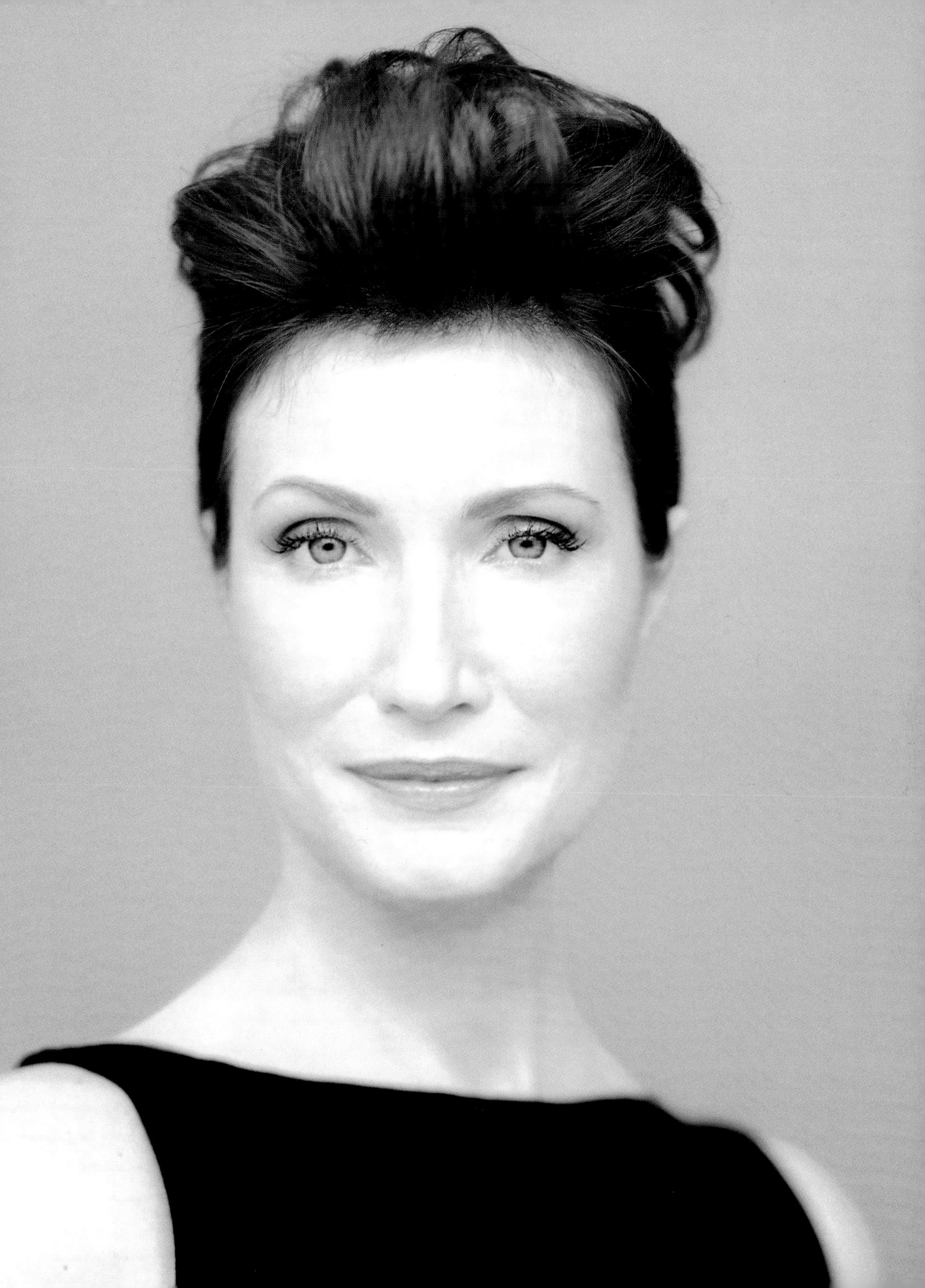

Model: Margaret Seymour. See Appendix C for specific makeup shades used in this photo.

refined glamour

You don't need a lot of makeup to look glamorous — just think of Grace Kelly. Here, Daniela is just wearing enough makeup to make her eyes stand out, and everything else is kept soft. This kind of soft, beautiful makeup always looks great and is easy for everyone to wear.

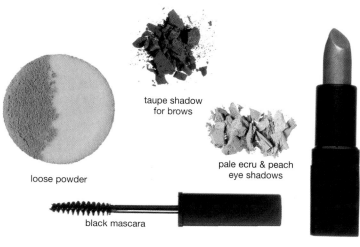

taupe shadow for brows

loose powder

pale ecru & peach eye shadows

black mascara

sheer iridescent pink lipstick

pink/bronze creamy makeup stick

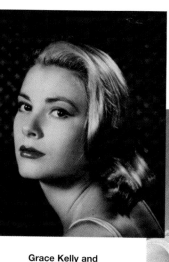

Grace Kelly and Catherine Deneuve — icons of refined makeup

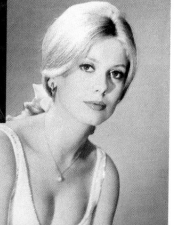

It's always pretty to use makeup only to enhance, where you'll say, "She looks great," not, "Her makeup looks great." This makeup look is still very natural, but defined just enough — and against Daniela's light hair and skin, the emphasis on the eyes and lashes is striking but not too strong.

Naturally Glamorous

1. Concealer was applied under the eyes where needed.

2. Foundation was mixed with moisturizer to sheer it down and smoothed over skin in a downward-and-outward direction.

3. To emphasize the skin and keep a dewy finish, creamy makeup stick in a pink/bronze shade was blended onto the areas the sun would naturally hit: forehead, tip of nose, and chin, with the most emphasis on cheekbones.

4. The brow was intensified with taupe powder shadow applied with an angled brow brush.

5. Black eye pencil was used on the outer three-quarters of the upper lid and then topped with dark brown powder shadow to blend. The shadow was swept outward and then down to line the outer third of the lower lid; everything was blended with a cotton swab.

6. Two pale eye shadows were used to shape the eye: a light ecru all over the lid and a slightly darker peach shade in the crease.

7. Several coats of black mascara, combed well between coats, were used on upper and lower lashes.

8. Loose powder was used on the forehead, nose, and chin only.

9. Lips were finished with sheer, iridescent pink lipstick.

1

5

5

6

7

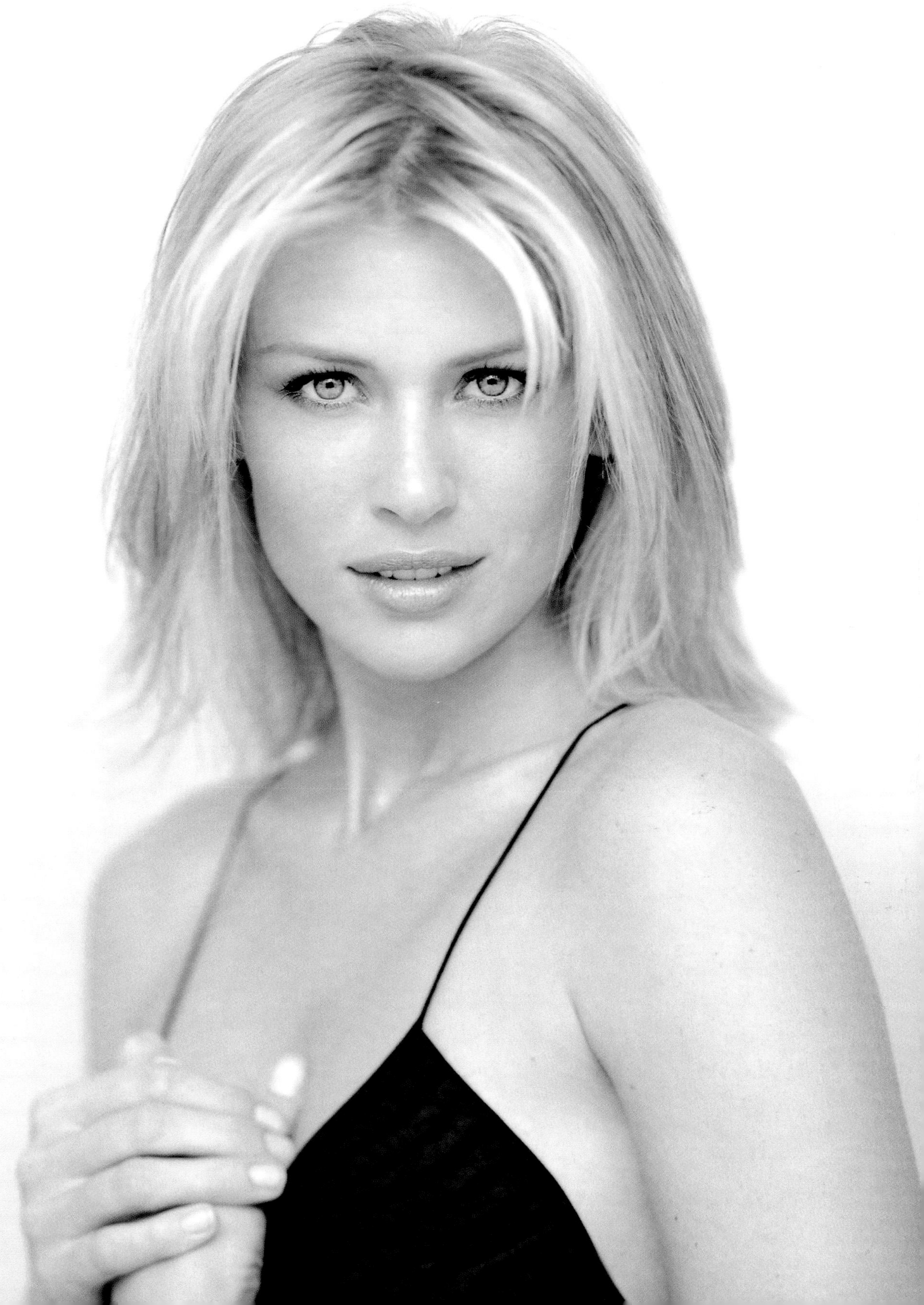

Model: Daniela Pestova. See Appendix C for specific makeup shades used in this photo.

timeless beauty

Older women often think that they need to wear brighter makeup, but that's simply not true. Carmen has a sophisticated look, but the colors are kept neutral and natural. To vary this timeless look, use less eye shadow and find a range of lip colors that work for you.

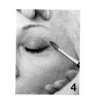

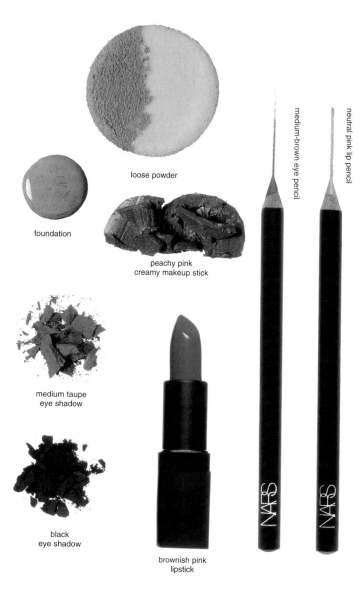

foundation

loose powder

peachy pink creamy makeup stick

medium-brown eye pencil

neutral pink lip pencil

medium taupe eye shadow

black eye shadow

brownish pink lipstick

NARS

NARS

black mascara

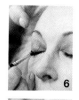

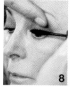

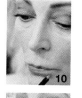

Less makeup looks better than more when you have older skin, so you have to refine your makeup skills — use just enough foundation and powder to even out your skin tone, apply color with a light hand, and blend everything very, very well so that it's as natural as possible.

Timeless Makeup

1. Concealer was used to correct darkness at the inner eye and around the mouth and nose.

2. Foundation was applied to the entire face and blended with gentle strokes.

3. A creamy makeup stick in a peachy pink shade was used to give cheeks a natural-looking glow.

4. A medium taupe eye shadow was applied wet all over the lid and then blended down when dry.

5. Medium-brown eye pencil was used to fill in sparse eyebrow areas, and then taupe shadow was blended over it with a shadow brush to soften.

6. Black eye shadow was used wet to line the top and bottom lids, with the line kept very close to the lashes. When dry, it was blended to soften and brought up a little at the end of the eye.

7. Dark taupe eye shadow was used all along the crease and blended upward.

8. Lashes were curled and then finished with two coats of black mascara on upper lashes only.

9. A little loose powder was applied to the forehead, nose, and chin to control shine.

10. Lips were lined with a neutral pink lip pencil to help lipstick stay in place; then a sheer coat of brownish-pink lipstick was applied with a brush.

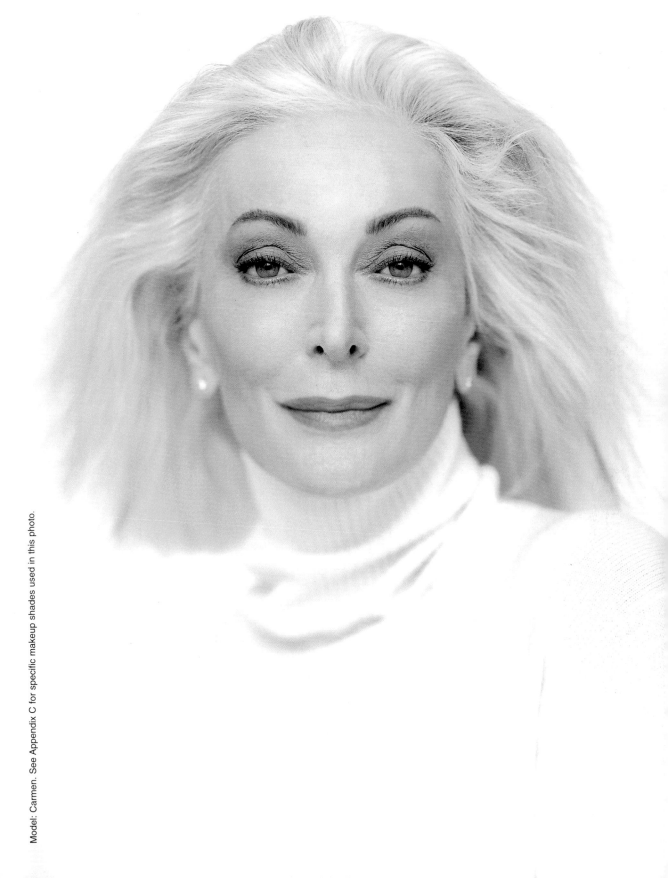

focus on skin

Nothing is more beautiful than gorgeous skin. It almost becomes a statement in itself: Because you have nothing to hide, you can get away with the bare minimum and still look great — a little enhancement here and there is all you need.

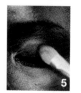

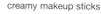

creamy makeup sticks

bronze   gold

Raquel's makeup (below) is about as easy as it gets — just two products — but it really plays up her skin, so it actually looks better than bare.

Simply Great Skin
1. A bronze creamy makeup stick was blended onto the chin, forehead, and cheeks — areas of the face that the sun would naturally hit.

2. The same bronze makeup stick was applied to the eyelids for added depth.

3. A shimmery gold creamy makeup stick was applied to the tops of the cheekbones, brow, top of the nose, and the ridge of the upper lip to highlight the face.

4. Both makeup stick shades were blended together with a lip brush and used as lip color.

When you want a more defined look but still want your skin to be the focus, it's just a matter of balancing your eyes and lips with your skin tone. If you have very light skin, you keep everything pale — and if you have dark skin like Margareth (right), you can use very deep shades.

Beautifully Balanced
1. Concealer was used around the eyes, nose, and mouth to lighten dark areas.

2. Two shades of foundation were mixed together for a precise skin-tone match, and applied sparingly all over the face.

3. A creamy bronze makeup stick was applied from forehead to temples, on the cheekbones, and along the jawline to highlight and bring dimension to the face.

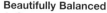

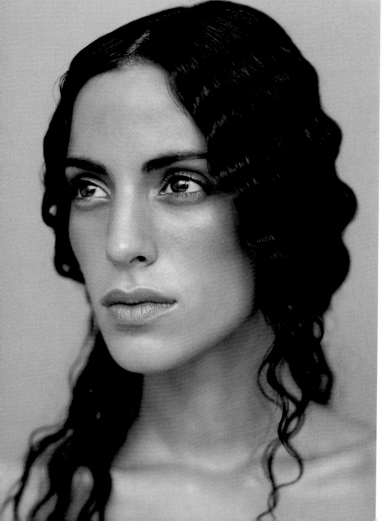

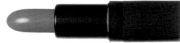

concealing stick

deep plum lipstick

4. Black eye pencil was applied to the eyes' inner rim, all over the lid, and along the upper and lower lash lines — then smudged all the way around the eye.

5. Black eye shadow was stroked on with a shadow brush to set pencil color in place.

6. Loose powder was used on the center of the face only to help matte shiny areas.

7. Deep plum lipstick was applied with a lip brush and then smudged with a fingertip for a more natural look.

two foundation shades were mixed

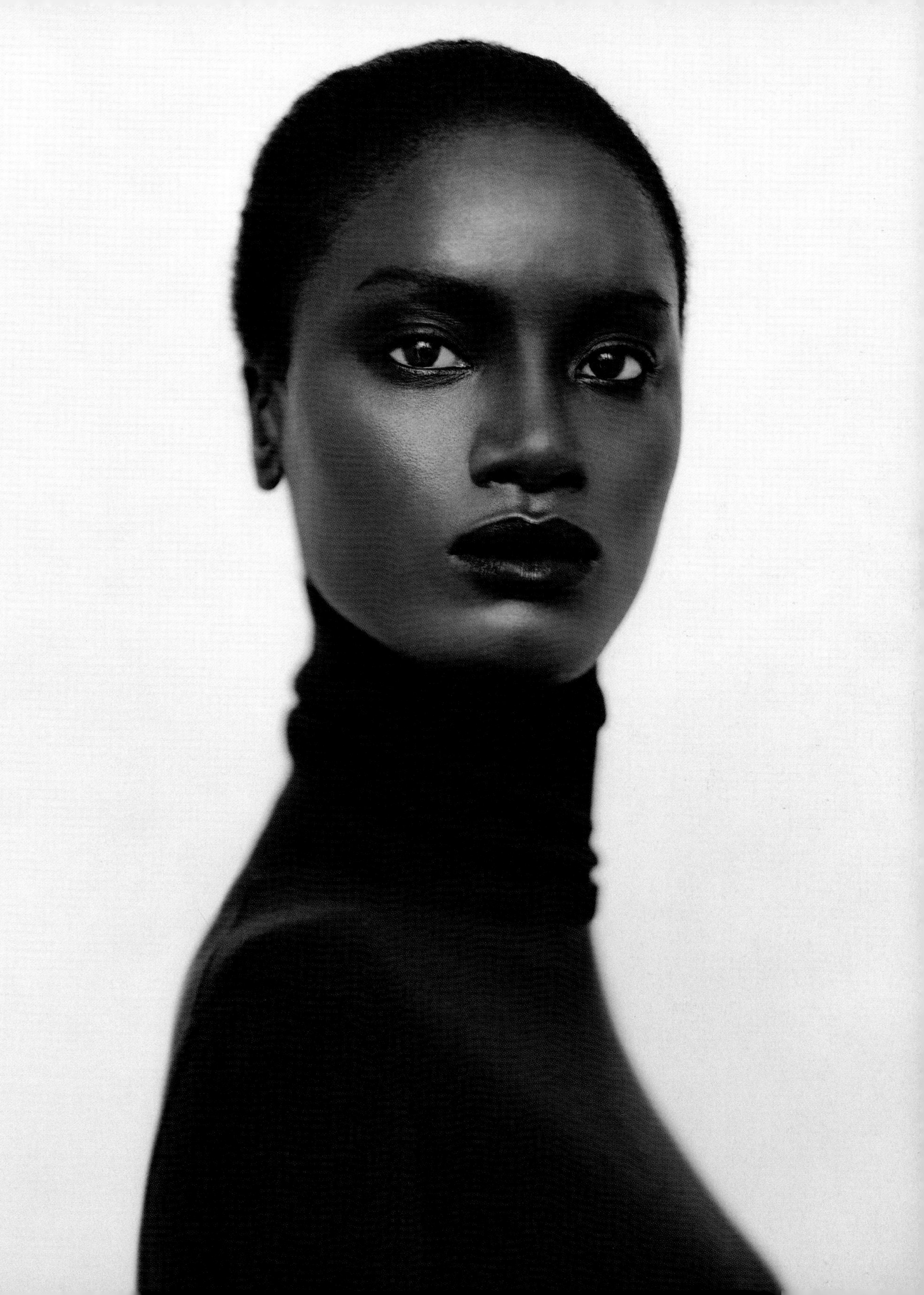

Models: Raquel (left) and Margareth (right). See Appendix C for specific makeup shades used in these photos.

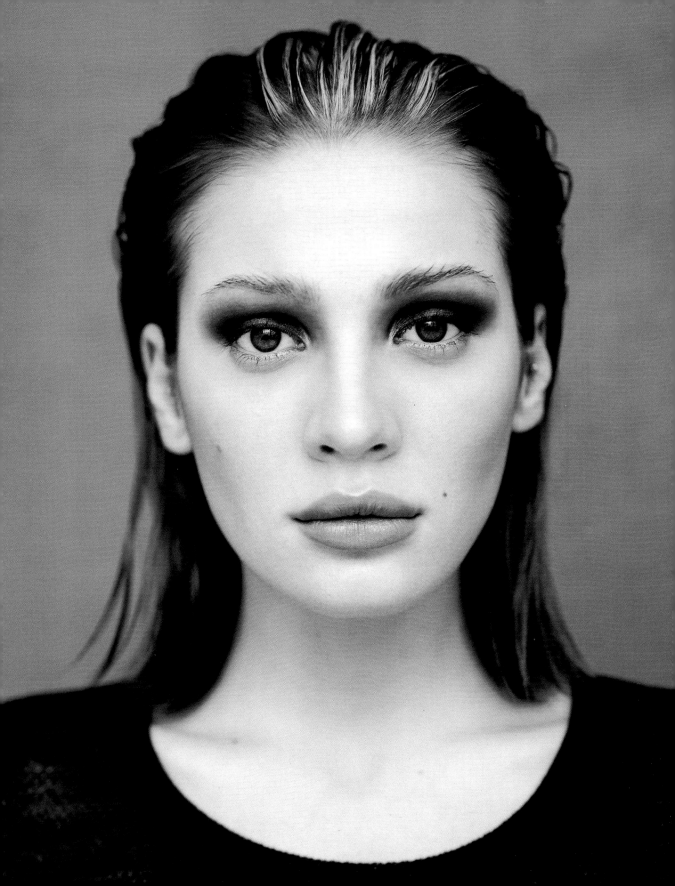

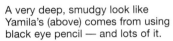

A very deep, smudgy look like Yamila's (above) comes from using black eye pencil — and lots of it.

Strong Smolder

1. Concealer was used under eyes where needed.

2. Pressed powder was dusted over the skin with a brush and then pressed into the face with a clean puff to give skin a satiny finish. Because Yamila had a tan, no blush was needed. If you want color on your cheeks, cream blush or powder bronzer works best.

3. To keep the look very natural, brows were brushed into place but no color was added.

4. Cobalt blue pencil was used to line the inner rim of the eye.

5. Black eye pencil was applied over the blue pencil; eyes were squeezed shut to smudge the color together.

6. The black pencil was applied to the top and bottom lids in a thick line and then smudged with a brush to give an almond shape to the eye.

7. Copper and brown eye shadows were blended together and then brushed on from lid to crease to blend and set the pencil in place.

8. Several coats of black mascara were used on top and bottom lashes.

9. Lip balm was used to give lips a moist look without adding color.

eye shadows

brown   copper   pearlized gray   black   charcoal

cobalt blue eye pencil

black eye pencil

focus on eyes

I've always loved the look of a dark, smoky eye — it's just so sexy and glamorous. The trick is to find your own version. Few women can wear that heavy Bardot black, but anyone can smudge on a little dark pencil or shadow and look dramatic. Blend everything very well and wear pale lip color so that your eyes really stand out.

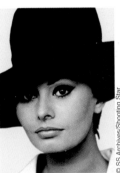
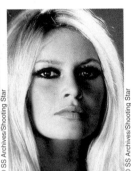

© SS Archives/Shooting Star

Divas of the dark eye: Sophia Loren and Brigitte Bardot

Eye shadow is a softer option for creating a deep eye. On Tatjana (left), all color was kept on the top lid only, and for a more modern look, no eyeliner or mascara was used.

Soft Smokiness

1. Concealer was used under the eyes and on flaws.

2. Brows were brushed up to groom; no color was added.

3. Pearlized gray eye shadow was brushed over the entire lid to give the next colors something to glide over and to give them dimension.

4. Black eye shadow was applied all over the lid up and into the crease, just meeting the inner and outer ends of the eyebrows.

5. Charcoal gray eye shadow was applied from the crease up and blended well with a brush.

6. Muted brown blush was brushed low on the cheekbones to give definition without "blush" color.

7. Sheer, neutral beige lipstick was applied with a finger for a soft look.

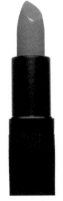

neutral beige (a peach or pink lip color with a neutral pencil adds color and definition)

focus on lips

When you really want to emphasize your lips, red is the ultimate. It worked for Marilyn Monroe — but you don't have to be a blonde bombshell to pull it off. With so many different shades and ways to apply them, every woman can find a red that's right for her.

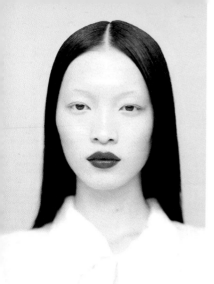

Model: Ling. See Appendix C for specific makeup shades used in these photos.

Wearing dark color on your lips doesn't have to be a big production. You don't have to wear lip liner if you don't want to, and you can apply the lipstick with your finger so that you just get a pretty stain of color. The key is to still have the feeling of lips — not lipstick.

Rethinking Red

1. Concealer was spot-applied to correct skin imperfections.

2. Foundation was used only where needed to even the skin tone and hide redness — important when wearing red lipstick.

3. Little dots of black eye pencil were applied between lashes to help them look thicker and then smudged until almost imperceptible.

4. A pale shade of pink eye shadow was applied to the entire lid up to the browbone.

5. Brows were brushed, but the color left natural; a filled-in line

pale pink eye shadow

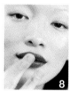

would have been too stark against a bold mouth.

6. Lashes were curled and given two coats of black mascara.

7. A medium pink blush was applied to the apples of the cheeks to give a healthy-looking glow.

8. Lip pencil was used to lightly define the border of the lips (particularly important if you have an irregular lip shape); then red lipstick was applied with the fingertips. Lips were then blotted with tissue for a softened effect.

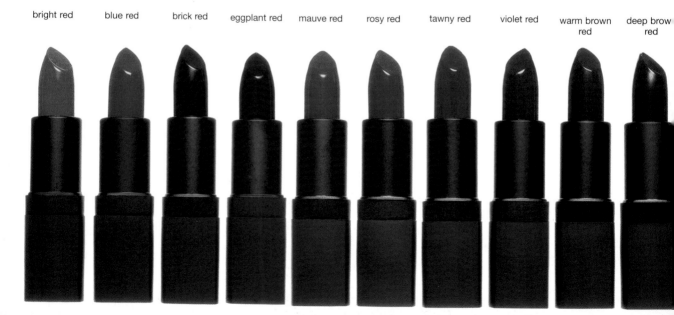

| bright red | blue red | brick red | eggplant red | mauve red | rosy red | tawny red | violet red | warm brown red | deep brown red |

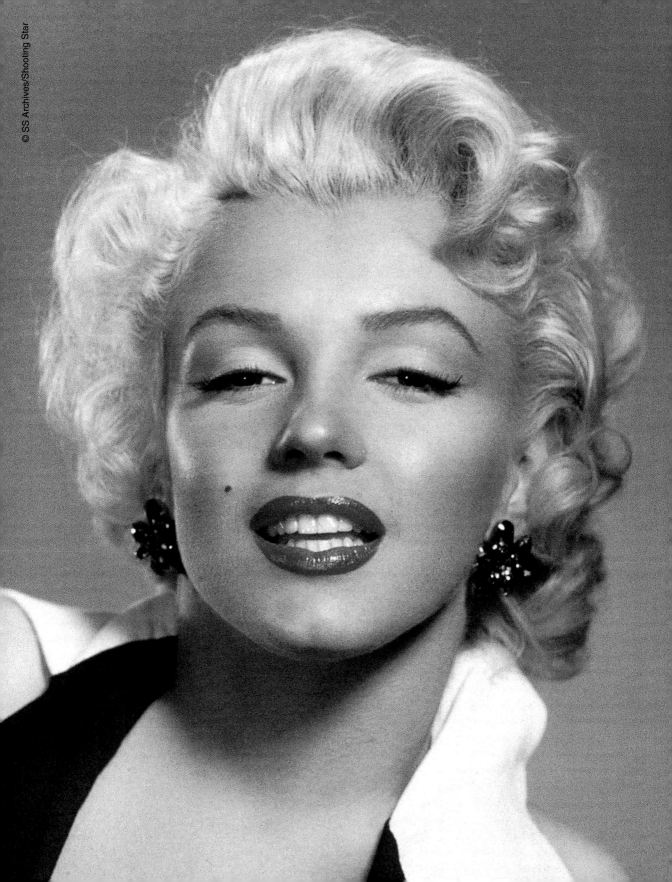

great shades

Neutral, natural colors like the ones shown here are the most versatile in makeup — in fact, the shades you see below are the actual Nars makeup used throughout this section. This palette of neutral tones works beautifully for any woman, any age, any skin tone.

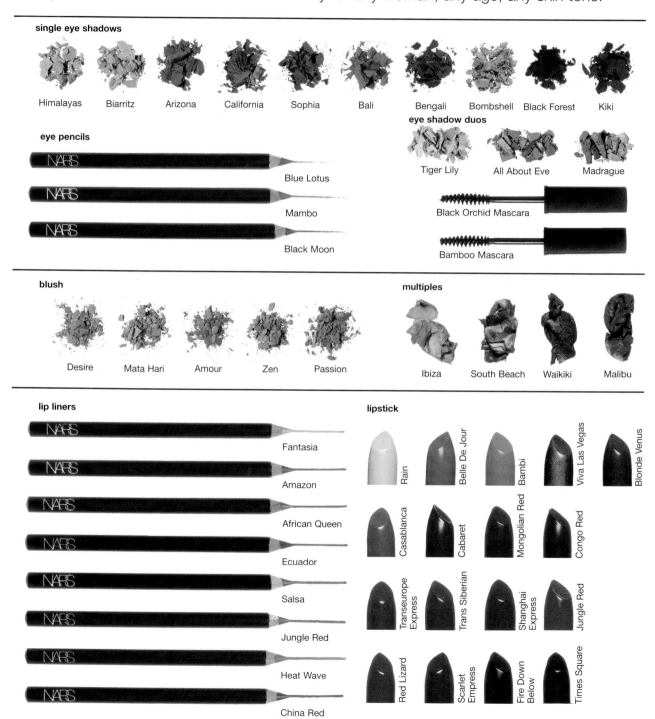

single eye shadows

Himalayas   Biarritz   Arizona   California   Sophia   Bali   Bengali   Bombshell   Black Forest   Kiki

eye shadow duos

Tiger Lily   All About Eve   Madrague

eye pencils

Blue Lotus

Mambo

Black Moon

Black Orchid Mascara

Bamboo Mascara

blush

Desire   Mata Hari   Amour   Zen   Passion

multiples

Ibiza   South Beach   Waikiki   Malibu

lip liners

Fantasia

Amazon

African Queen

Ecuador

Salsa

Jungle Red

Heat Wave

China Red

lipstick

Rain   Belle De Jour   Bambi   Viva Las Vegas   Blonde Venus

Casablanca   Cabaret   Mongolian Red   Congo Red

Transeurope Express   Trans Siberian   Shanghai Express   Jungle Red

Red Lizard   Scarlet Empress   Fire Down Below   Times Square

Chapter 12

Gathering Your Tools

• •

In This Chapter

▶ Determining which brushes and accessories you really need

▶ Organizing your makeup

▶ Setting up your workspace

• •

The right tools are what *really* separate the finger-painters from the Picassos. They make all the difference in how your makeup goes on and how it looks after you apply it.

Assembling Your Toolkit

You need full-sized, well-made brushes in order to get the most from your makeup. You can find them anywhere makeup is sold: drugstores, department stores, beauty supply shops. A good brush is a good investment, so go for the best quality you can afford. With proper treatment, a quality makeup brush will last for years.

Just because a manufacturer included a brush with your blush or eye shadow does not mean that it's up to the task. These small items are usually made from inexpensive materials that don't hold or blend color well.

When choosing your brushes, keep these points in mind:

✔ Look for natural-hair bristles that feel soft and smooth (bristle content is usually printed on the brush handle). Reject any brush that sheds or has a splayed, messy head.

✔ Test bristles on your skin to see whether they're firm enough to place color with precision, yet not so stiff that they'll scratch or pull during application.

> ✔ Make sure that the handles are rounded and smooth, comfortably tapered, and long enough to rest easily in your hand.
>
> ✔ Stay away from premade sets. Buying each brush separately is a better bet — that way, you pay only for what you'll really use.

Art supply stores are a great resource for finding a wide range of high-quality brushes at reasonable prices. If the handles are too long for you to use comfortably (or pack easily), remove a few inches with a small saw and sand the end smooth.

The essentials

Figures 12-1 and 12-2 show photographs of some must-have brushes and other essential tools. Use these photographs and the tips in this section as a guide when purchasing your own set of makeup tools.

If you really want your makeup to go on right, six brushes are indispensable. That number may seem a bit excessive at first, but each brush is made for a specific task and can help you do your makeup quickly and easily. After you see the difference these brushes make, you'll wonder how you ever survived without them.

> ✔ **Powder brush:** Wide and fluffy, this brush is the largest of the group, made to dust loose or pressed powder evenly over the skin.
>
> ✔ **Eyeliner brush:** You use this thin, flat brush to place and blend color near the lash line.
>
> ✔ **Eye shader:** Used to apply powder color on the eyelid, this flat brush has either a rounded or an angled shape.
>
> ✔ **Eyelash separator:** Made for combing out clumps and other mascara blunders, this brush helps lashes look natural and soft. You'll find many types — wire, plastic, spiral (like a mascara wand) — so choose whatever works for you.

> The eyelash separator is also commonly found combined with an eyebrow brush (see "The extras," later in this chapter) in an all-in-one tool. The spiral eyelash separator (which resembles the business end of a mascara wand) works well for both purposes, too. In fact, an old mascara wand, thoroughly cleaned with eye makeup remover, does the trick for both lashes and brows.
>
> ✔ **Blush brush:** Soft and medium-full with a rounded shape, this brush blends powder color evenly over the cheeks without streaks or stripes.

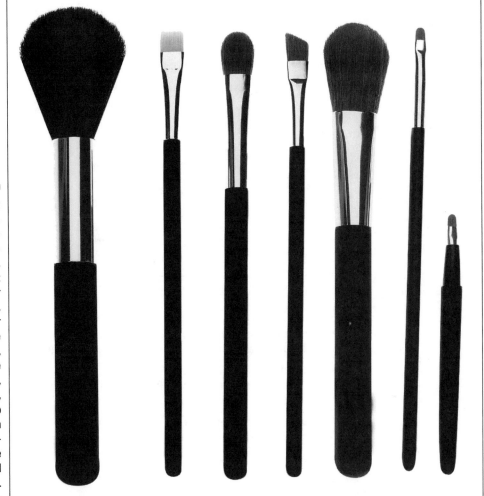

Figure 12-1:
The indispensable makeup brushes, left to right: powder brush, eyeliner brush, eye shader, angular eye shader, blush brush, and lip brush (both non-retractable and retractable).

✔ **Lip brush:** A lip brush is flat and slightly tapered to glide around the mouth's curves and place color precisely. This brush is essential for applying deep-toned lipstick and mixing one or more lipstick shades together to create your own color. A covered, retractable type is handy for throwing in your purse or makeup bag.

These items aren't brushes, but they're essential all the same:

✔ **Tweezers:** You just can't skimp on this tool. Buy the best set of rust-proof, stainless steel, precision tweezers you can find. (Tweezerman is the favorite among makeup artists.) Take good care of them: Dropping them or throwing them into a travel bag unprotected can dent the tips and render them unusable. Here's the rundown of tweezer types:

Figure 12-2:
From left to right: three types of eyelash separators, pointed-tip tweezers, slant-tip tweezers, scissors, pencil sharpener, traditional eyelash curler, and corner eyelash curler.

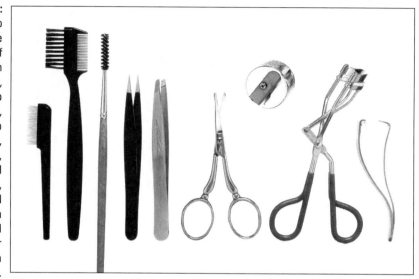

- **Slant-tip tweezers** are good generalists that can see you through most plucking scenarios.

- **Pointed-tip tweezers** are the most precise; good for snagging fine and just-emerged hairs. Resist the urge to dig, and use this tool carefully.

- **Square-tip tweezers** tend to remove too many hairs at once; I recommend that you pass on these.

- **Round-tip tweezers** are pretty much worthless, except for applying individual eyelashes. Don't bother.

✔ **Scissors:** Small, round-tipped scissors are great for trimming overly long brow hairs and visible nose hairs.

✔ **Pencil sharpener:** It sharpens pencils.

✔ **Eyelash curlers:** If your lashes are straight, these tools add a bit of curl and help open up the eye area. You'll find a couple of different types, both of which usually come with extra pads:

- The classic curls the entire row of lashes.

- You can also get spot-curling devices known as *corner curlers.* These are used mainly for curling the outer corners of the eyelashes, which a full curler has a hard time getting to. They come in a variety of sizes and are harder to find — try a specialty drugstore or beauty supply shop. A corner curler is indispensable for giving the lashes an upturned effect.

Your eyelash curler must fit your eye comfortably. If it isn't wide enough, you won't be able to curl your entire row of lashes. Many different designs are available, so find one that you can use with ease and that accommodates your lashes.

TIP

Keeping it clean

If you give your brushes the proper care, they'll give you years of loyal service. Clean them every couple months if you use them daily — less frequently if you use them less often (although storing them clean is a good idea). Overzealous cleansing can be just as harmful as lack of care, so take it easy. Here's the proper way to do it:

✔ Wet brushes with warm water and then gently work a drop of mild soap (such as Ivory) into the bristles with your fingertips. Don't smash or splay the bristles while sudsing; you'll break the hairs and ruin the brush's shape.

Some beauty supply stores and drugstores carry special cleaning solutions made to dry-clean makeup brushes. Frankly, they're no more effective than soap, and they can contain undesirably harsh chemicals. Save your money.

✔ Never leave a brush soaking in water; you'll cause the bristles to come unglued, and the metal fittings may rust.

✔ Rinse the brush thoroughly under a running tap and then gently press out the excess water with a towel.

✔ Reshape the bristles into place and then let them air-dry by laying the brushes flat with their heads hanging over the edge of a table or countertop so that air can circulate on all sides.

If a brush's bristles become splayed, don't continue to use it: You'll get imprecise application. Wash the brush, use the tiniest bit of hair gel if necessary to train hairs back to where they should be, and let the bristles air-dry. The next time you use the brush, check your technique; grinding the brush into the product — or your face — is probably the source of the problem. Ease up.

While you're working on your brushes, take a few moments to do a little upkeep on your other makeup tools:

✔ Wipe tweezer and scissor tips with alcohol to remove oil build-up that can cause the tools to slip.

✔ Wash sponge-tip applicators, eyelash curlers, powder puffs, and non-natural bristle brushes (such as a brow color brush) in soap and water. Press out any extra moisture and let them air-dry.

✔ Replace anything that sheds, shreds, or otherwise falls apart.

The extras

Depending on your preferences, your needs, and your choice of makeup products, you may want to add some of the following brushes to your toolkit:

- ✔ **Eyebrow brush:** This brush helps you blend brow-color products and grooms the brows into place.

    You can also groom your brows with an ordinary toothbrush — just not the one that you use on your teeth!

- ✔ **Brow color brush:** This stiff, angled brush with synthetic bristles is used to blend powder color at the brow; it can also be used to blend brow pencil. If you need daily color fill-ins as opposed to just a brush-up, this brush is a smart purchase.

- ✔ **Concealer brush:** If you have a scar, a birthmark, or uneven pigmentation that needs correction on a regular basis, you may want an extra brush expressly for concealer. Using a brush helps you place cover-up exactly where it's needed. Two basic types of brushes exist: One has a very thin, pointed head for placing color precisely on small areas; the other is flat, with a firm texture and a small, tapered head for blending color over larger areas, such as under the eye.

- ✔ **Liquid eyeliner brush:** This brush, which has very few, short, fine bristles, enables you to draw a very precise line. Liquid eyeliner is a bold look that's not for everyone, but if you wear it, this brush is a must-have for proper application.

The helpers

Disposable and indispensable, these staples are a must to have on hand:

- ✔ **Cotton swabs:** You can use them as-is for blending, dampen them for repair work, or pull off their little cotton heads and use the sticks to dig out the last lipstick from a tube. The good ol' classics work just fine, although the new ones that are flat on one end and pointed on the other are highly recommended by professional makeup artists for perfecting and cleaning up the edges of eyes and lips or for applying eye shadow in a pinch. (See Figure 12-3.)

- ✔ **Sponge-tip applicators:** Using these tools (also shown in Figure 12-3) is also a matter of personal preference. Although sponge-tips can grab too much color, making them less than ideal for applying shadow to the lid, they do come in handy for blending powder shadow over eye pencil to help smudge and set color.

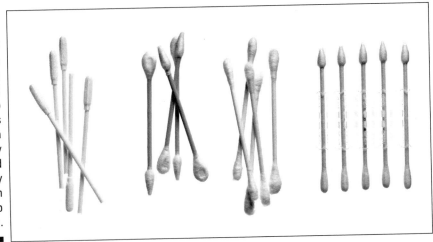

Figure 12-3:
Cotton swabs and sponge-tip applicators come in a wide variety of types and have many uses in makeup application.

✔ **Makeup sponges:** Your options include flat and wedge shapes (as shown in Figure 12-4) as well as natural sea sponges — the type you choose is a matter of personal preference. Although fingers can't be beat for applying foundation and concealer, a dampened sponge can come in handy for blending creamy products after they're on your skin. However, sponges tend to absorb a great deal of product, and latex versions can cause allergic reactions in some women.

✔ **Powder puff:** Made of cotton velvet or velour, a puff can help you press powder firmly into your skin for more staying power or to give it a more matte finish. (See Figure 12-4.)

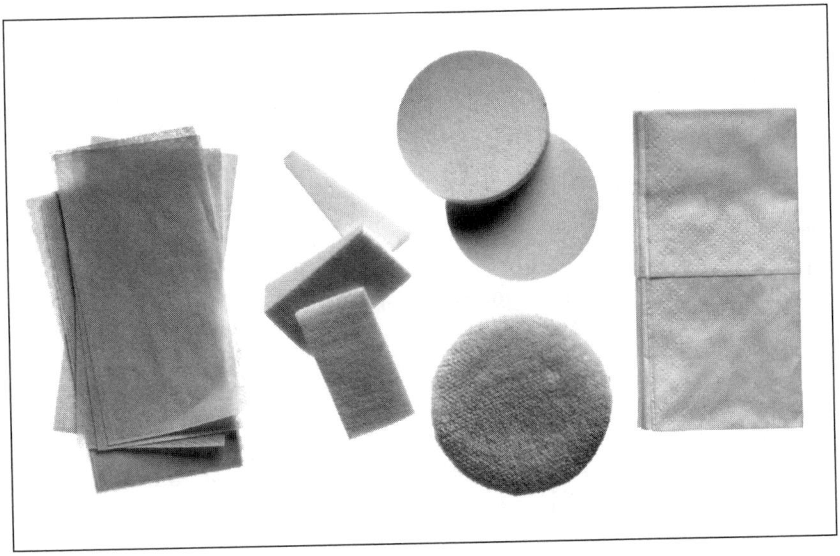

Figure 12-4:
Blotting papers, makeup sponges, powder puffs, and tissues are indispensable makeup tools.

- **Tissues:** These little wonders, also shown in Figure 12-4, blot lipstick to a more matte finish, absorb excess oil from the skin, and buff away excess facial powder.

- **Blotting papers:** Similar to tissues, these papers are used to blot away excess oil and makeup. (See Figure 12-4.)

Getting Organized

An important part of making makeup work for you is being sure that it's ready when and where you need it. When you're in a rush, your makeup can't be scattered all over the place — not only will you be aggravated and flustered, but you may *never* find the mascara or blush you want to use. You'll save yourself a lot of time and frustration if you keep everything ship-shape on a daily basis.

Makeup bag

Ideally, you should have two makeup bags: one that contains all the products you use regularly, and another for the extra fun stuff, such as bronzer, colors that you don't wear every day, and so on. Make sure that your everyday bag is small enough to throw in your purse or tote bag and washable so that you can keep it looking neat. You should be confident that it contains everything you need — and nothing you don't — so you're never stuck with the wrong product at the wrong time.

- Some products (such as foundation and loose powder) aren't necessary to take along on a daily basis unless you wash your face during the day.

- If you work in an office, keep duplicate makeup in your desk drawer to eliminate the need for carrying makeup back and forth.

- Go through your everyday bag often to see whether it contains anything you haven't been using. Retire that product to your extras bag, or toss it if you know that you'll never use it again.

- Most makeup artists pop the blush, eye shadow, and other color pans out of the individual packaging and attach them (using glue or double-sided tape) to a box that's specially designed to hold several palettes of makeup. You can create your own personalized version by purchasing a box (available from Make Up For Ever and other manufacturers) that holds all your makeup products in one place. You can even make two boxes: one with the essentials and one with the extras. Or try a compartmentalized container to tote all your different shades of lipstick. By using these tricks, you instantly eliminate most of your makeup bag clutter.

Makeup area

As you may know from trying on foundation, viewing your makeup in real daylight is *the* way to check for a natural look — therefore, applying your makeup by natural light only makes sense. I realize that the architecture of your bedroom, bathroom, or office may make this feat impossible, but you *can* at least check your look by the nearest window after your makeup is on.

Fluorescent light is the absolute worst light for making-up in; incandescent is better; full-spectrum light bulbs give a truer color read. Whatever your light source, try to have it hit your face evenly. Anything too harsh or beaming sharply in from above distorts your perception.

Work in an area that gives you plenty of room for spreading out your makeup and tools: You can't concentrate on what you're doing if things keep teetering off the sink edge and crashing to the floor. Some women store their products on a tray in the closet; others have a makeup table or vanity just for the purpose. Simply figure out what works best for you.

TIP

Makeup clean-up

Every makeup bag needs a spring cleaning every now and again — it's a great way to take stock of what needs to be replaced and what should be retired. Just dump it all out on the counter and have at it: Toss anything that's irreparably broken. Stash away in your extras bag anything you haven't used lately. All the rest should get a good cleaning — putting on your makeup is always more inspiring when it's clean and organized.

✔ Clean bottles and tubes with a tissue or a cotton pad soaked in alcohol or non-oily makeup remover.

✔ Dust around powder eye shadow and blush pans with a cotton swab dampened with alcohol or water.

✔ Sharpen makeup pencils (clean out the sharpener with a cotton swab after each use). If your pencils are very soft, freeze them for about an hour to firm them before sharpening.

✔ Clean compact mirrors with a cotton pad soaked in alcohol.

✔ Wash application sponges or powder puffs with mild soap, use a towel to press out the excess water, and let them air-dry. Or simply replace them with new ones (which you can find at most drugstores).

✔ If you notice that a hard, shiny film has formed on the surface of a powder product, scrape it off. That film is simply facial-oil build-up; the product beneath is perfectly fine to use.

✔ Wash your makeup bag to get rid of all the smears and bits of makeup inside. Throw it in the washing machine (if it's fabric) or soak it in the sink with a little soap.

My mother's bathroom is a perfect lesson in organization. Under her sink, she has a great little organizer on wheels. It's aluminum with four or five narrow mesh baskets, and it holds all her makeup, hair brushes, hair products, and blow-dryer — her whole beauty regimen, all in one spot. The baskets even lift out, so she can put them on the sink when she's doing her makeup or hair and have everything right there.

Chapter 13

Shaping Your Brows

*W*hat do eyebrows have to do with makeup? Everything. They're your face's most changeable feature — they give you personal style and can completely change the look of your face. Shaping your brows can make your eyes seem bigger, smaller, closer-set, or farther apart, which realigns the entire balance of your face. This chapter shows you how.

Brow Basics

Staying with your natural brow shape usually looks best — don't ever try to alter your natural arch. After you create the shape that's right for your eye, your face, and your style, use makeup to enhance the arch and play with the brow's shape. Adding or subtracting a little bit is perfectly fine; just be aware of the effect that it will have on your face. In general, a thicker brow is considered softer and more youthful, while a thinner brow shape can make you look harder and older.

All those pencil-by-the-nose tricks aren't really necessary, although you can use a pencil to measure if you're not sure of yourself. Remember these simple guidelines (also see Figure 13-1):

✔ The brow should begin in line with the inner corner of the eye. The line doesn't have to be precise — in fact, it looks better on some women to leave the inner edge a bit inexact.

✔ Never try to change your brow's natural arch by tweezing — you'll ruin the shape of your brow.

✔ The brow should fade out gradually beyond the eye's outer corner.

✔ The brow's width should taper only slightly from beginning to end.

✔ The beginning of the brow should never be lower than the end of the brow; you'll look like you're scowling.

✔ The end of the brow should not dip lower than the outer corner of your eye; if it does, it drags your eye down.

Simple, huh?

Figure 13-1:
Brows should start in line with the eye's inner corner and fade gently toward the eye's outer corner, with both ends at approximately the same level.

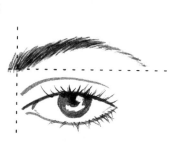

Finding Your Best Brow Shape

Keeping the basic guidelines in mind, you can customize certain eye types a little bit more:

✔ If your eyes are **close-set,** you may want to take a little more from the inner part of the brow to help create the illusion of width. A few hairs may be all that's necessary, so don't overdo. (See Figure 13-2.)

✔ If your eyes are **wide-set,** begin the brow a little closer toward the nose to visually pull your eyes toward the center of your face; you can also remove a little from the brow's outer end. Again, it may just be a matter of a few hairs on either end of the brow; check your look after each pluck. (See Figure 13-3.)

✔ If your eyes are very **small,** removing weight from the bottom of the brow helps to open up more lid area, creating the illusion of a bigger eye. (See Figure 13-4.)

Figure 13-2: Brow shaping for close-set eyes.

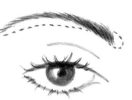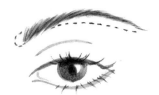

Figure 13-3: Brow shaping for wide-set eyes.

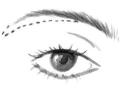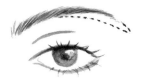

Figure 13-4: Brow shaping for small eyes.

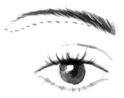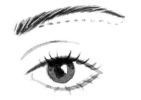

Undesirable shapes

Undesirable shapes often occur when you make an eyebrow tweezing mistake. People even have names for them — The Tadpole (as shown in the figure at right), The Toothbrush, The Hook, The Comma. All these brows are considered unbalanced and extremely unflattering. See "Brows 911" later in this chapter to find out how to grow and reshape your brow into a more flattering shape.

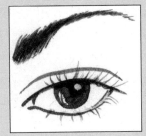

Tweezing Tipsheet

✔ If you'd rather not shape your brows yourself, have someone do it for you. Many hair salons, day spas, and beauty centers offer brow-shaping services. Although waxing is the most common method, some places tweeze as well. After that, you can maintain the shape yourself by tweezing away what grows back. Remember to express what you do and don't want. Pictures can help you express yourself.

✔ Tweeze eyebrow hair after a shower or bath; your skin is softer and your pores are more open, allowing hair to slide out easier. Or place a warm washcloth over your brows for five to ten minutes before tweezing to achieve the same results.

✔ Gently exfoliate the brow area with a scrub or washcloth to help free any trapped hairs (doing so daily helps to prevent those nasty stuck-in-there hairs).

✔ If you have a low pain threshold, apply a topical anesthetic (like Anbesol) before tweezing.

✔ A good way to preview a new brow shape is to "erase" hairs before you actually remove them. Use a white nail pencil, pencil-form concealer, or concealer on a small-tipped brush to "white out" hairs; if you're happy with the look, tweeze only the "erased" hairs — one at a time, of course.

✔ Tweezing brows in natural light is optimal.

✔ Don't wear eye makeup while tweezing. Because eye makeup visually reshapes the eye, you won't be able to judge the work to be done as accurately — and the makeup is also likely to smear or run.

✔ Use the best tweezers possible. I recommend Tweezerman tweezers (see Appendix B for contact information).

✔ Pull your skin taut and remove hairs — one by one, not two or more at a time — in the direction of growth.

✔ Grasp hair close to the root and pull gently. If you grab the hair by the end, not only do you have to pull harder — which can break off hairs near the root rather than removing them cleanly — but you're also needlessly pulling the skin.

✔ Plucking a hair does *not* cause it to grow back thicker; if anything, tweezing hairs may stop hair growth altogether.

✔ No matter what brow-shaping method you use, go slow and recheck often; a tweezing mistake can take three to six months to grow back. Remember, you don't have to do it all in one day, so take your time — and stop if you feel unsure.

> ✔ Never tweeze hairs from above the brow; you'll ruin your natural arch. If you have very dark, fine hairs that aren't part of the brow proper, bleach them instead to give the brow area a cleaner look (see "Other Brow Shapers," later in this chapter).
>
> ✔ Close your pores with astringent after tweezing.

Brow Tweezing Step-by-Step

Brow shaping is serious, so give yourself plenty of time to relax and do it right. Don't feel that you have to complete *all* the following steps. Though you should follow them in order, you can stop after completing any one of them if you're happy with the way your brows look. Keep in mind that the inner corner and the arch give the brow its shape, so focus on these areas as you tweeze, continually visualizing the brow shape you want to achieve.

1. **Get rid of obvious renegade hairs, including hairs that grow down onto the eyelid, between the eyes, or past the outer end of the eyebrow.**

2. **Define the inner corners, plucking hair by hair until the brow's inner edge is in line with the eye's inner corner.**

   Try to avoid tweezing an unnaturally straight, vertical edge: You're better off leaving some hairs that fall slightly outside the line. Repeat with the other brow.

   Remember to pay attention to the individual quirks of each eyebrow. No two eyebrows are alike. Strive for balance rather than perfection.

3. **Working from the inner corner to the outer corner on the underside of the brow, thin out overly thick areas by removing one hair at a time until all the hairs in that row are gone (see Figure 13-5).**

   Leave any hair that falls slightly above that row; you'll get a softer effect and avoid leaving holes. While tweezing, remember to brush your brows back into place often so that you can see exactly what you need to remove. When brushing your brows into place, groom them in the direction of their natural growth.

4. **Bring your other brow into balance by removing hairs one by one as in Step 3.**

   After you remove one row of hair from each side, rebrush your brows into place and then stand back and scrutinize your work from a distance. If you need to do more, repeat Steps 3 and 4.

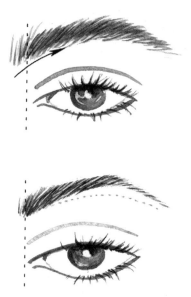

Figure 13-5:
Tweeze
hairs one
by one,
working
from the
eye's inner
corner
outward.
Avoid a too-
straight
inner edge
by leaving a
few hairs
outside
the line.

If you're not sure about removing a certain hair, leave it alone. You don't have to be exact with the shape. Leaving it is always better than regretting it later. After a few days, you'll know whether the hair was meant to be there.

Brows 911

I know how easy it is to get tweezer-happy. Here's the method I've used to regrow my brows after making tweezing mistakes. It was passed along to me by makeup artist François Nars (who also photographed and designed the looks for the Makeup Workbook section):

1. **First of all, expect total regrowth to take three to six months.**

   Not what you wanted to hear, but it's true; some hairs may not be in a growth phase and will take a long time to reappear.

2. **Use an eyebrow pencil to fill in your brows to the shape you *want them to be.***

   Make sure that your pencil is sharp and not greasy — you want fine, hair-like strokes, not a thick blob of color.

3. **Tweeze any hairs that fall outside that ideal shape.**

    If you're not sure about tweezing something, leave it alone. When more hairs fill in, you'll be able to tell what stays and what goes.

    If you have trouble keeping yourself from plucking, give your tweezers to a friend for safekeeping while you're trying to regrow. To pacify yourself, keep your brows well-groomed by brushing them into place.

Don't be alarmed if some brow hairs grow back in strange directions — they should straighten out eventually. In the meantime, brush them into place with a little brow gel or hairspray. Some hairs may never reappear. Repeated plucking can kill the hair follicle, which means that it's not coming back . . . ever.

Other Brow Shapers

Altering the look of your brow is not limited to tweezing, though that's the most overwhelmingly popular method. Here are some other recommended options:

- ✔ **Waxing:** Offered by many hair and beauty salons, waxing is a great way to create an initial shape for your eyebrows if you aren't confident in tweezing. After waxing, all you need to do is keep up the shape. Although I love the cleanliness and shape that waxing gives to the eyebrows, I usually break out from waxing. If you have very sensitive skin like I do, be cautious of waxing on your face.

- ✔ **Bleaching:** If your brows are markedly darker than your hair, if they grow untamed above your arch, or if you just want the face-softening effect of a lighter brow color, you can bleach your eyebrows yourself. Use a gentle facial hair bleach (the stuff made for the upper lip) and leave it on for two minutes. Make sure that the consistency is on the thick side — you don't want this stuff running or dripping into your eyes. Wipe away gently, carefully rinse with water, and then brush your brows back into place and let them dry. If the hair's still too dark, repeat a day later, again for two minutes. If you feel any burning, itching, or discomfort at any time during the process, remove the bleach immediately and thoroughly flush the area with water.

    Brunettes beware: Too much bleach on the eyebrows will look red.

- ✔ **Dyeing:** The official line on brow (and lash) dyeing is that it's simply not done, although I think that both can be very necessary, particularly for those women with pale eyelashes or eyebrows that need enhancing due to hair coloring. Always consult a professional when it comes to eyelash or eyebrow dyeing. If you have any questions about your eyebrows while coloring your hair, ask your hair colorist. Many salons that give facials also dye eyelashes.

Snip snip

Tweezing is not the only solution for shaping brows — you may only need a trim. Overly long brow hairs can give brows a bushy, overgrown appearance, but if you remove the hairs entirely, you can be left with holes. To give your brows a teeny little haircut, follow these steps:

1. **Brush brows straight up and then snip anything that's obviously too long with small, round-tip scissors.**

   Don't go all in a straight line; snip to different lengths to keep the line from getting harsh or straight.

2. **Brush brows straight down and then trim any excess.**

3. **Brush brows back into place. Carefully snip any hairs that are still too long, going one by one and brushing between each snip.**

   Don't cut them all the same length or try to form them into a line; the result will look unnatural. Random is best.

Don't cut it too close. Though grow-out doesn't take as long as with tweezing, regrowing a too-trimmed hair can take a month or more. Start with little snips; then do more only if needed.

Chapter 14
Applying Your Makeup

· ·

In This Chapter

▶ Step-by-step application techniques
▶ Corrective techniques

· ·

*A*fter you get your formulas and colors right, it's time to put them to work. Applying makeup is fun, but it's also a skill where practice certainly does make perfect. Have fun, and remember: It washes off.

Applying the Essentials

Nine key makeup products are used to create a variety of looks: foundation, concealer, powder, brow color, eye shadow, eyeliner, mascara, blush, and lip color. You don't have to use them all at once — some items you may *never* use, depending on your makeup style — but you should always have the essentials on hand so you know that you're ready for anything.

There are no rules to makeup application. Combining my personal techniques with your own should give you as many looks as you choose to create with the most personal effect. Keep in mind that makeup is an illusion; it doesn't have to be perfect. I try to do it as perfectly as I can, but I don't spend hours trying to get every little detail right.

I personally have plenty of makeup looks that I know look good. They're all basic but simple: A smoky eye and a pale lip. Mascara and a red mouth with a rosy cheek. But I like to play like anybody else. I've never done my makeup one way all the time. I have this big pile of makeup — people give me products all the time — and depending on where I'm going and what I'm doing, I just do whatever I'm in the mood for. I don't even wear makeup every day.

Before you start applying your makeup, look at your face with no makeup on and ask yourself honestly, "What do I want to change?" With me, my eyelashes droop down in the corners — I like to curl them so that my eyes turn up a little. I have a few holes in my eyebrows and they're uneven, so I balance them out with brow color. When I'm pale, I look good with a little blush. It's all about looking in the mirror and saying, "What do I like about my face, and what can I make better?" Use makeup to make changes to satisfy *yourself.*

Makeup application tipsheet

✔ If you don't feel comfortable wearing lipstick, or foundation, or *anything,* don't force yourself. You'll look as uneasy as you feel.

✔ Don't try to dramatically redraw your face with makeup. Simply enhance your best qualities and try to play down the rest.

✔ Do most of your hairstyling before applying makeup. After makeup's complete, give your hair a quick once-over and you're ready to go.

✔ Tailor your makeup to what you're doing that day. Going to the park with friends? Don't automatically put on your office face. A little concealer and lip balm may be all you need.

✔ It's always better to underapply than overapply. Adding more color is easy — and removing it can be tricky.

✔ Play, play, play with your makeup, and have fun experimenting with new things. Feeling timid? A great time to try something different is at night: You'll feel more relaxed when the light — and the mood — are more low-key.

Foundation

The first step to applying foundation is to scrutinize your skin. Look closely in the mirror and really notice what's going on with your face before you start your makeup. You may be having a Bad Skin Day and decide that you want extra coverage. Or maybe your skin looks fabulous and you feel like skipping foundation altogether. Small changes occur in your skin every day, so don't get stuck doing the same old, same old simply out of habit. I recommend using a sheerer coat of your foundation or a tinted moisturizer during the day and giving yourself a bit more coverage in the evening.

Applying foundation

1. **On a clean face, apply a thin layer of moisturizer all over the face and under the eyes.**

2. **Place a small amount of liquid or cream foundation on your finger-tips and begin to apply it evenly all over the face and undereye area. Gently pat it in and make sure that there are no obvious streaks or lines.**

   If you prefer to use a sponge, make sure to use a clean one each time, or wash the one you use regularly to make sure that the foundation goes on as thin as possible.

3. **Check your hairline and jawline for lines of demarcation and blend well with dampened fingertips or a sponge.**

   If you're not using concealer, you can apply your powder now.

Foundation tipsheet

✔ For the smoothest-ever foundation application, exfoliate your skin first, and then moisturize any areas that feel tight or look flaky. If you're applying moisturizer or sunscreen to your entire face, let it absorb into your skin for about ten minutes before applying foundation.

✔ As an alternative to foundation, try tinted moisturizer. It gives the most natural-looking coverage and usually comes with an SPF.

✔ If you have dark skin, avoid any foundation or sunscreen that contains titanium dioxide. This ingredient can give darker skin an ashy appearance.

✔ If you feel that your skin needs extra coverage, apply two thin coats of foundation rather than a single heavy layer — it looks more natural.

✔ When you need the coverage of full-face foundation, you can make it look more natural by blotting some away from your cheeks and nose. Your natural skin tone shows through, giving the impression that you have less makeup on your face.

✔ Foundation should be absorbed into the skin, not sit on the surface. If it looks too thick, lightly spray your face with water or dampen your fingers and then continue to blend.

✔ Foundation can be used on eyelids and lips to prep the palette, getting rid of any discoloration, and also works as a fix-it, keeping your lipsticks and eye shadows truer longer.

Concealer

I always apply my concealer after my foundation. That way, the concealer covers anything that the foundation doesn't. However, if you're not wearing foundation, concealer should be your first step. There are different techniques for applying concealer, depending on what you're trying to hide. I've broken it down into two sets of steps: The basic technique is for the undereye area, and the other is for correcting blemishes, scars, veins, undereye puffiness, freckles, and other types of discoloration.

Applying concealer: The basics

1. **If you haven't already moisturized your undereye area, apply a thin layer of moisturizer and let it absorb into your skin.**

2. **Get a small amount of concealer on your tiny concealer brush or your ring fingertip.**

3. **Lightly brush in two directions or pat with your ring finger from the inner eye outward, continuing out as far as needed and focusing your attention on areas of discoloration.**

   You don't want to put concealer lower than the bone under your eye.

4. **Blend with your ring finger all over the undereye area, starting from the outside and working your way in.**

   If you're powdering, powder now. If you're not powdering and you're planning to wear eye makeup, make sure to use a drier form of concealer or your eye makeup will smear.

Applying concealer: Corrective techniques

More serious flaws require specialized techniques. If you have an area that needs extra help on a daily basis, you'd be smart to invest in a heavier concealer formula that's made for lasting, opaque coverage. You also need a separate concealer brush to apply it (see Chapter 12). Fingers are good for blending, but they're not the right tool for precise placement.

- To spot-apply concealer onto a **pimple** or **spider vein,** use a small, thin concealer brush to apply it directly where needed. You may need to lightly pat in the concealer with your fingertip. Make sure that your concealer is not too light, or it will only make a raised blemish stand out more.

- To help correct **undereye puffiness,** blend concealer on the darker, recessed area *under* the puff, not on the puff itself. The lighter color helps "raise" the darker area to even out the eye area's look. You might also want to try a cooling eye gel five to ten minutes before applying your concealer.

- To help correct **scars,** you need to use an adherent concealer formula because scar tissue tends to be very smooth. With your brush, blend the concealer evenly onto the scar and set with powder.

- To help correct **hyperpigmentation** (including age spots, port-wine stains, and melasma, or "mask of pregnancy"), apply your foundation first and then lightly brush on concealer, being careful to stay within the border of the darker area. For more intense coverage, you may have to apply a second layer. Finish with a light dusting of powder.

Concealer tipsheet

✔ Be sure to apply concealer to the eye's inner corner where the eye meets the nose — doing so makes your eyes look brighter and more rested.

✔ Be careful not to overapply or use a color that's too light — you'll get a "reverse raccoon" look.

✔ To get extra coverage, use two thin layers of concealer only where needed.

✔ Concealer can help even out darker pigmentation over large areas of the face: around the mouth, on uneven patches on cheeks, and over melasma. Apply with your fingertip, using a light patting motion, *before* foundation's on.

Powder

Powder is the makeup miracle worker. If you're using a creamy or liquid foundation, powder sets it in place; if you're using other powder-form makeup, powder helps it to glide easily and evenly over the skin — and also works as an eraser if you've applied too much. But before you disappear in a puff of powder, remember that a little shine is normal on healthy skin. If you overpowder, you'll erase your own natural skin tone, leaving your skin looking lifeless and overly made-up.

Applying powder

1. **Dip your powder brush into loose powder, tap off the excess, and dust lightly over the face.**

2. **Take a close-up look at your skin in the mirror; if powder is obvious in your fine facial hairs, continue to blend with your brush, puff, or fingers until everything looks smooth.**

Powder tipsheet

✔ Pressed powder can be also applied with a brush — simply swirl the bristles until they loosen and pick up enough powder, tap to remove any excess, and whisk onto the face.

✔ If your foundation and powder seem too heavy, simply blot with a tissue or washcloth moistened with a bit of water, or spray water onto the face with an atomizer and reblend.

✔ When you're not in a powder mood but still don't want shine, try special blotting papers made for absorbing facial oils (available in most drugstores).

✔ To keep foundation from collecting in facial creases, use only as much product as necessary, blend it very well into the skin, and then "set" it with loose powder. Finish by blending or blotting with a velour puff.

✔ If shine is a problem that the occasional powder touch-up doesn't seem to remedy, you may want to change your foundation and/or moisturizer. Overpowdering only makes your skin look dry and cakey.

Eyebrows

Once you've shaped your brows (see Chapter 13), they're ready to be filled in with brow color (if needed) and brushed into place.

Applying brow color

1. Using your eyebrow brush, groom hairs in the direction of growth to reveal the natural line of the brow and to find the areas where fill-ins are needed.

2. For **basic shaping and filling with color,** you have two options:

   • **Powder color:** Gently pat the end of your angled brow color brush into the powder, tap off any excess, and then stroke onto the brow where needed. Finish by blending the color and grooming the brows back in place with your brow brush.

   • **Pencil color:** Lightly stroke hair-like lines onto bare spots, as shown in Figure 14-1, and then use your brow brush to blend the color and brush the brows into place. A little powder brow color or loose powder helps the pencil color stay put.

Figure 14-1:
Brow pencil strokes should be fine and hair-like, following your brow's natural growth pattern.

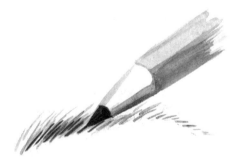

For **major brow redrawing,** use a sharp, firm-textured pencil. Fill in bare areas with small, hair-like strokes, as shown in Figure 14-2, using your real hairs as a guide for the direction of your pencil strokes. Resharpen the pencil as you go; then set color in place with a very light dusting of loose powder.

If there's next to nothing left of your real brow, use your brow *bone* as your guide. Feel the area above your eye with your fingertips to find where your forehead meets your eye socket: Most brows fall right on that ridge, so that's where you want to apply color.

Figure 14-2: If you have no brow hairs left, use your brow bone to guide color placement.

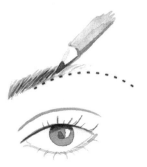

Eyebrow color tipsheet

- ✔ Stay within the parameters of your natural brow to get the most flattering effect. Work on a soft, natural arch and be careful with the inner part of the eyebrow — it should have the softest color.

- ✔ If you're wearing major eye makeup that extends from the outer corner of your eye, extend your brow a little, too — doing so keeps everything in balance.

- ✔ Don't use brow color if you don't really need it; sometimes brushing the brows into place is enough. To help keep brow hairs in line, use a clear brow gel or a little hairspray or styling gel on your brow brush.

Eye shadow

Applying eye shadow can be as quick and easy as applying one color on the entire lid or as involved as using two or three colors for a more sophisticated effect. Here are the steps for a classic three-shade application; for more specific instructions on maximizing your personal eye shape, see "Shaping eyes with color" later in this chapter.

Applying eye shadow

1. **Using your eye shadow brush, sweep your medium-toned shadow all over the lid.**

   If all you want to do is to give the lid a clean, natural appearance, stop after this step.

2. **With the same brush, use your darker-toned shadow to define the eye's crease.**

   You can also use this shade, wet or dry, to line the eye by using your eyeliner brush (see the instructions later in this chapter).

3. **With your lightest-toned shadow, highlight the brow bone or center of the eyelid if desired.**

Eye shadow tipsheet

- ✔ If you're going for a very dark eye, take a tip from makeup artist Glenn Marziali: Do your eyes entirely before moving on to the rest of your face. If shadow scatters, you can just wash it all off instead of making spot-repairs.

- ✔ For smooth, even eye shadow application, prep your lids with a thin layer of foundation. If you're using a cream eye shadow and have problems with creasing, use concealer first and then top the eye shadow with powder.

- ✔ Keep the basic principles of light and dark in mind as you apply color: Darker colors make areas recede, while light color brings them forward.

- ✔ For easiest application, start with the shadow shade that goes over the most eye area (usually your medium tone) and then work your way down.

- ✔ If you're using an eye shadow pencil, don't draw directly onto the lid — you'll stretch and pull the skin. Instead, swatch a circle of color into the palm of your hand, swirl your fingertip in the color, and then apply the color to the lid.

- ✔ When using colors that are definitely outside the neutral palette, stick to one shade swept over the eye rather than several.

Eyeliner

Because eyeliner products are so different in texture and create such different effects, you need to know the steps specific to the product you're using. Here, I give you the basic application steps for each type of eyeliner. Choose the right type of liner for the effect you want: Liquid draws on intense, sharp-edged color; pencil gives a smudgier effect; shadow creates a very soft line. For more specific techniques for maximizing your eye shape with eyeliner, see "Shaping eyes with color" later in this chapter.

Lining the inner rim of the eye

If you're going to use your eyeliner to line the inner rims of your eyes, make sure to use a freshly sharpened pencil (only pencil works here); a fresh surface lessens the chance of introducing bacteria into the eye. For the lower lid, place a finger below the lower lid and gently pull downward to better expose the surface. For the upper lid, pull up the eyelid to expose the inner rim. Then carefully glide the pencil along the rim.

Applying pencil eyeliner

Your pencil has to have the right tip if you want to get a good line. Here's a great trick that I've picked up from watching makeup artists work: Sharpen your eye pencil and then lightly scribble with it on the back of your hand. Doing so helps dull down that very sharp point and warms the tip so that it's gentler on the skin. And those little clumps that break off from the tip land on the floor, not your face.

1. **Gently pull the lid skin taut and, starting at the inner eye, glide the pencil smoothly along the upper lid, getting as close to the lashes as possible. One swoop or several little connected dots will do.**

2. **With a small eye shadow brush, blend the line from the inner lid to the outer lid. Doing so softens the line, refines the desired eye shape, and softens the color.**

3. **If you want to line the lower lid as well, use a light hand to trace a gentle line of color near the lashes.**

4. **Gently smudge the liner under your eyes with a small eye shadow brush.**

Applying shadow eyeliner

Using eye shadow to line your eye is smart for lots of reasons: It saves having to buy a separate product. It saves space in your makeup bag. And it's the most versatile liner option you have: You can use it dry for a very soft line; or, as done here, you can use it wet for more intensity and staying power.

1. **Wet your eyeliner brush and work it into your powder shadow.**

2. **Test color intensity and texture on the back of your hand, and use more or less water if necessary.**

3. **Close your lid, gently pull the skin taut with your finger, and sweep color along the upper lid, getting as close as possible to your lashes.**

4. **Line the lower lid, if desired, again staying close to the lashes.**

5. **If color or shape is less than perfect, use your flat eye shadow brush to blend and soften the line after the shadow has dried completely.**

   Still too harsh? Use the same brush to tone things down with a little loose powder.

Applying liquid or cake eyeliner

Liquid eyeliner is quite difficult to apply, so it's a good idea to get organized up front. First of all, make sure that your brush isn't damaged or splayed. Second, moisten a few pointed cotton swabs with a little eye makeup remover before starting your eyeliner application and keep them handy. They help non-pros get professional-looking results.

Liquid liner should be applied before anything else. If you have to start all over, you won't ruin the rest of your makeup.

1. **Test for color, intensity, and sharpness of line by applying liner to the back of your hand.**

   If you're using cake eyeliner, wet your eyeliner brush and work it into the cake first.

2. **Close your eye and pull your eyelid taut with your fingertip.**

3. **Starting at the inner corner of your upper lid, pull the eyeliner brush in a straight, even line as close to your lashes as possible. (See Figure 14-3.)**

   If that's too hard for you to do, try doing a connect-the-dots or connect-the-dashes approach. Just take it slowly and don't panic.

   If you go past the lashes, the line should curve up rather than down.

Figure 14-3:
Apply liquid eyeliner from the eye's inner corner outward, as close to the lashes as possible.

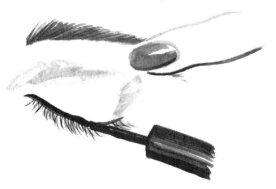

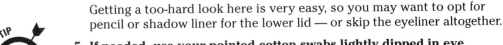

4. **For the lower lid, turn the brush vertically to get beneath the lashes and apply liner very, very carefully.**

   Getting a too-hard look here is very easy, so you may want to opt for pencil or shadow liner for the lower lid — or skip the eyeliner altogether.

5. **If needed, use your pointed cotton swabs lightly dipped in eye makeup remover for shaping and perfecting the line.**

   This trick works great for women who love that cat-eye effect but have a difficult time perfecting it.

Eyelining tipsheet

✔ Take the edge off a too-harsh line with loose powder or powder shadow blended on with your eye shadow brush.

✔ If you're using pencil, make sure that the texture is right: too hard and you'll pull delicate lid skin, too greasy and it'll end up smearing under your eyes.

✔ Get liner right next to your lashes to make them look thicker, and check to make sure that you leave no bare spots. A thin strip of skin between liner and lashes is not attractive.

✔ Never line the lower lid only. Doing so drags down your eyes — and your entire face — and makes you look ever so sad.

Mascara

The great thing about mascara is that it's so versatile. One coat gives you a natural effect; two coats give you a thicker, more dramatic look; and three coats give you an intense, "spidery" effect. Always start with one coat and continue until you've achieved the desired effect. Several coats of mascara will need combing through.

Applying mascara

1. **If desired, curl your lashes with a regular or corner curler to open up the eye area. (See "Working the Extras" later in this chapter for instructions.)**

2. **To get mascara all the way down to the lash roots, which makes lashes look their thickest, place a finger mid-lid or on your eyebrow and pull up.**

3. **Holding the wand horizontally, sweep on mascara from roots to ends; roll the wand slightly as you move along the lashes to distribute mascara evenly (see Figure 14-4).**

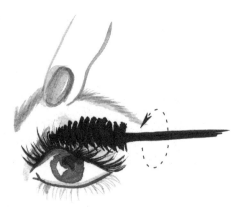

Figure 14-4:
For best
mascara
application,
pull the lid
slightly
upward
and roll the
brush to
coat lashes
evenly.

4. **Using your spiral brush or lash comb, give lashes a brush-through after they've dried to remove any clumps and give the lashes a more natural look.**

5. **If you want mascara on your lower lashes, hold the wand vertically and lightly sweep across the lashes or go lash by lash.**

According to makeup artist Glenn Marziali, "Most women can skip mascara on the lower lashes altogether. It really doesn't do much for defining the eye and almost always ends up smudging."

Mascara tipsheet

✔ If you're wearing a rich eye cream or concealer, your mascara will end up under your eyes. Try a less-emollient concealer or change your undereye moisturizer, and remember to powder lightly to prevent smudging.

✔ If your lashes aren't as lush as you'd like after the first two to three coats, try switching mascara formulas. Thickening formulas do work.

✔ For the most natural mascara effect, wipe the mascara wand with a clean tissue to remove excess product before applying.

✔ To build optimal thickness, be sure to let mascara dry completely between coats.

✔ If your lashes are very light, you may want to apply mascara to the top side of lashes as well so that you don't have two-toned lashes when you blink.

Shaping eyes with color

As explained earlier in "Applying eye shadow," the classic approach to maximizing eye shape uses three eye shadow shades — light, medium, and dark. The medium shade serves as the base color and can range from quite pale to really deep, depending on the look you want to create. After you choose your medium shade, you can figure out how intense the other two should be. The dark shade is commonly known as *contour color;* the lightest is called the *highlight shade.* These two shades help create the illusion of depth and projection, respectively, when applied to specific areas of the eye.

For truly corrective eye shaping, shadow should be followed with eyeliner and mascara. (Remember, you can also use your darkest shadow shade, wet or dry, as liner.) Skillful application of these eye makeup essentials can really bring your face into balance, and learning the techniques that work best for you isn't hard to do.

Find your eye shape or shapes in the following sections; then just follow along step-by-step. (Some people have combination eye shapes; for example, my eye shape is round but droopy at the corners. Combine the techniques as needed.) You may not do a full-on eye-shaping every day, but it's good to know the principles — and how to do a full eye-shaping when you want to look your absolute best.

Figure 14-5 labels the parts of the eye to help you as you go through the steps for your eye shape.

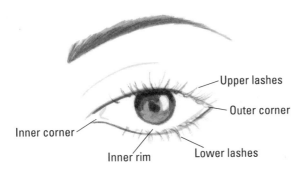

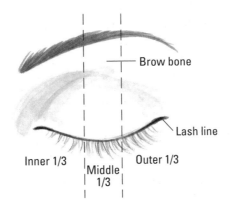

Figure 14-5: The parts of the eye.

Eye type: Small

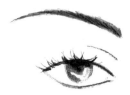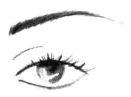

Objective: To create the illusion of more eye area by concentrating color on the outer portion of the eye

Shadow Steps:

1. Sweep medium-toned shadow on the upper lid and up to the crease.

2. Apply the contour shade at the outer third of the crease.

3. Add highlight just under your brow's arch.

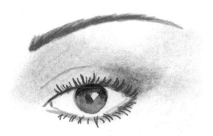

Eyeliner:

- *Upper:* Concentrate liner at the outer third of your upper lid. Blend up and out to extend the line, making sure that contour shadow and liner are blended together.

- *Lower:* Concentrate liner at the outer third. Blend up and out to extend the line.

Mascara: Use mascara on your top lashes, concentrating on your outer lashes. Use no mascara or a smaller amount for the bottom lashes.

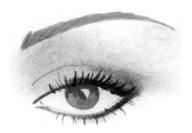

What Works:

> ✔ Keep your medium shadow shade toward the lighter end of the spectrum to help open up the eye.
>
> ✔ Keep eyebrows well-groomed to open up more eye area (see Chapter 13).

What Doesn't:

> ✔ Avoid dark shadow shades all over the lid; they give eyes a closed-in look.
>
> ✔ Be careful of lining the inner rim of the eye; it tends to make the eye look smaller.

Eye type: Round

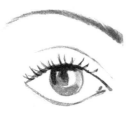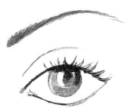

Objective: To lengthen the eyes' look by applying color with a more linear, horizontal emphasis

Shadow Steps:

1. Apply medium-toned shadow all over the lid.
2. Apply contour shade all along the crease, extending it slightly at the eye's outer corner.
3. Add highlight under the brow's outer third.

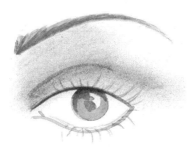

Eyeliner:

> ✔ *Upper:* Begin at the eye's inner corner, line the full length of the upper lid, and then extend outward and upward at the end. Use a corner curler to lift the outer lashes.

> ✔ *Lower:* An extremely light eyeliner, used only to enhance the lash line, is preferable under the eye.

Mascara: Use mascara on top lashes only, concentrating on the outer half of the eye.

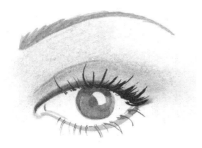

What Works: Keep color on the upper lid to "cut" the circle in half.

What Doesn't: If you're using an eyelash curler, try a corner curler rather than the traditional type. The traditional curler will only emphasize the roundness of the eye; a corner curler will give the illusion of length.

Eye type: Vanishing lids

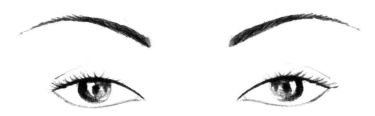

Objective: To create emphasis and depth, as the eye has no natural crease

Shadow Steps:

1. Sweep on medium-toned shadow from lash line to brow bone.
2. Concentrate the darkest shade just above the crease; then blend and fade toward the brow.
3. Add highlight on the brow bone.

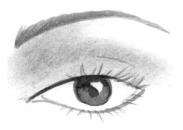

Eyeliner:

- *Upper:* Staying right at the lash line, sweep color on the outer two-thirds of the upper lid.
- *Lower:* If you wish, apply a very slight line under the lower lashes.

Mascara: Curl lashes first to open up the eye; apply mascara to top lashes.

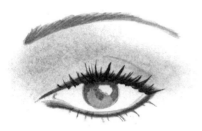

What Works:

✔ Stay with deep, neutral tones and blend well to avoid obvious lines.

✔ Keep eyebrows well-groomed and off the brow bone (see Chapter 13).

What Doesn't:

✔ Don't try to create a crease where none exists. Use contour color for enhancement.

✔ Heavy black eyeliner tends to close off the eye. If you're using cake or liquid liner, be sure that your lines are thin and precise. For tips, see "Applying liquid or cake eyeliner" earlier in this chapter.

Eye type: Deep-set

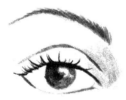 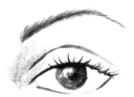

Objective: To de-emphasize the recessed look created by a deep natural crease

Shadow Steps:

1. Use medium-toned shadow over the entire lid.

2. Place contour color just above the crease and blend upward.

3. Add highlight under the brow bone.

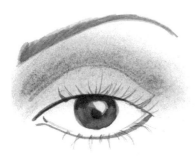

Eyeliner:

> ✔ *Upper:* Use a very light hand, keep color right at the lash line, and blend well.

> ✔ *Lower:* Use only to enhance the lash line, and blend well.

Mascara: Apply mascara to upper lashes and lower lashes, combing well between coats if you apply more than one.

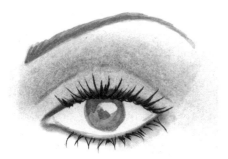

What Works: Keep shadow toward lighter shades to counteract the crease's darkness.

What Doesn't:

> ✔ Don't put contour shade right in the crease; the eye will only recess further.

> ✔ Avoid heavy eyeliner; it echoes the darkness of the crease and counter-acts your efforts to lighten the look of the eye.

Eye type: Close-set

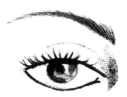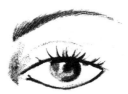

Objective: To create the illusion of wider spacing by emphasizing the outer portion of the eye

Shadow Steps:

1. Apply medium-toned shadow all over the lid.
2. Place contour shade at the outer third of the crease and blend outward at the outer edge of the eye.
3. Highlight the brow bone at the eye's outer third.

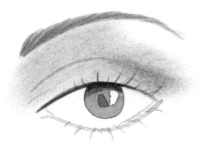

Eyeliner:

✔ *Upper:* Start about halfway across the upper lid and extend the line slightly past the outer corner; blend to soften.

✔ *Lower:* Line the lower lid from about the same point; blend to soften.

Mascara: Apply one coat to all lashes, and then a second on outer lashes only. If you use mascara on your lower lashes, use it only on the outer few.

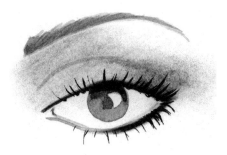

What Works:

✔ Keep color concentrated on the outer portion of the eye.

✔ Remove a few hairs from the brow's inner edge to open up the area (see Chapter 13).

What Doesn't: Avoid applying color to the inner part of the eye; you'll close it right back in.

Eye type: Wide-set

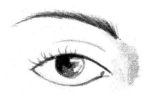 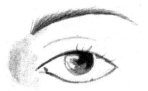

Objective: To create the illusion of closer spacing by emphasizing the inner portion of the eye

Shadow Steps:

1. Use a medium-toned shadow over the entire lid.

2. Apply the darkest shade in the crease from about midway on inward, blending into the hollow that reaches from nose to brow.

3. Highlight under the brow's arch.

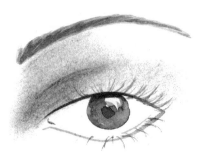

Eyeliner:

 ✔ *Upper:* Begin liner right at the inner corner, draw outward to the eye's outer third, and then blend the line to fade toward the outer edge.

 ✔ *Lower:* Begin liner right at the inner corner, draw outward to the eye's outer third, and then blend the line to fade toward the outer edge.

Mascara: Apply mascara to upper and lower lashes.

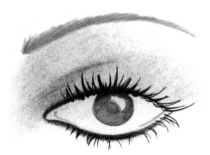

What Works:

 ✔ Keep color concentrated on the inner portion of the eye.

 ✔ Allow brows to grow in full at the inner portion of the eye, which visually draws in the eye (see Chapter 13).

What Doesn't: Never extend liner or shadow past the eye's outer corner; doing so only separates the eyes further.

Eye type: Downturned

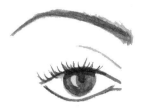 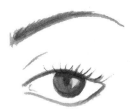

Objective: To visually lift the outer corners of the eyes

Shadow Steps:

1. Apply liner first in this case; then sweep a medium-toned shadow over the lid.

2. Place a contour shade in the crease, following the shape created by your eyeliner. Stop before contour and liner meet at the outer corner.

3. Highlight under the brow's arch.

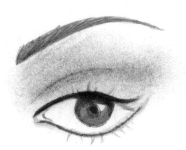

Eyeliner:

> ✔ *Upper:* Liner comes first here: Start the line at the eye's inner corner, follow your natural lash line until you reach the eye's outer third, and then pull liner across, sweeping it above and beyond the lash line.

> ✔ *Lower:* Draw a line that parallels the top lid's, sweeping it up at the end. Do not join the two lines.

Mascara: Apply to outer lashes only, right where liner begins to sweep upward. Use your corner curler to bring the corner lashes up.

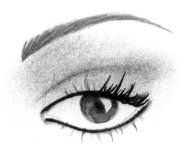

What Works:

- Keep color moving upward at the outer corners of the eyes.
- Try individual lashes at the corner of the eye. (See "Individual eyelashes" later in this chapter.)

What Doesn't:

- Don't follow your entire lash line with liner; you'll emphasize the downward droop at the end.
- Don't let liner get smudgy under the eye; it drags your eye back down.

Eye type: Mature

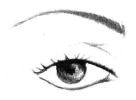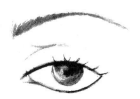

Objective: To de-emphasize lid crepiness and heaviness

Shadow Steps:

1. Sweep your medium shade over the entire lid.

2. Skip the contour shade; it's very difficult to place on less-than-supple skin.

3. Don't use a highlight shade under the brow unless your skin is taut.

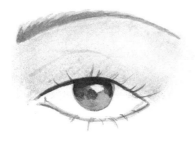

Eyeliner:

✔ *Upper:* Apply color along the lash line, with the line growing a bit thicker toward the eye's outer third. Blend well.

✔ *Lower:* Nothing at all is usually best.

Mascara: Not always necessary. If you use mascara, apply only one very light coat.

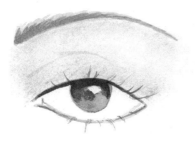

What Works: Neutral, subtle shades even out the look of the lid.

What Doesn't:

✔ Don't try to resculpt hollows where skin is no longer taut.

✔ Keep color away from areas that are very wrinkled; color calls attention to the flaw and can even settle into creases.

Blush

Have you noticed the conspicuous absence of "contouring" instructions in this chapter? Well, you won't find them here, either. Used on photo shoots and television to visually sculpt and reshape the face — most often the cheek area — contouring techniques really have no place in real life. So instead of trying to color-on new cheekbones for yourself, use blush to make the most of what you already have. For most women, that means applying blush on the apples of the cheeks for a natural, healthy-looking effect. As a rule, always start blush two fingers away from the nose and above the hollows of the cheeks, as shown in Figure 14-6.

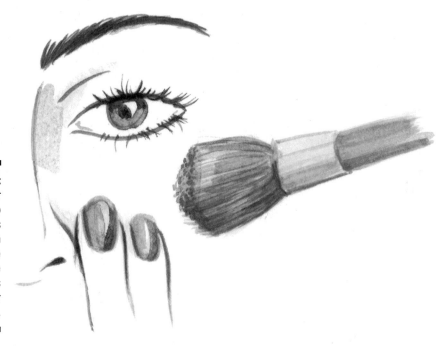

Figure 14-6:
Start your blush two fingers away from your nose and above the hollows of your cheeks.

Applying powder blush

1. **Lightly coat your blush brush evenly with color, tap off any excess, and then sweep the brush over the apples of your cheeks.**

   Not sure where your apples are? Look into the mirror and give yourself an exaggerated smile. The area that pillows up is what you're aiming for.

2. **Work the brush back toward your hairline, blending with both upward and downward strokes until you see no visible edge between blusher and skin.**

Applying cream blush

1. **Put a small amount of the product on your fingertips.**

2. **Lightly press your fingertips over the apples of your cheeks and cheekbones, blending the blush very carefully until it's completely absorbed into the skin.**

   A second application may be necessary.

3. **Tissue off any excess blush left on your fingers.**

Blush tipsheet

- ✔ If your powder blush is going on streaky, you may need to powder your cheeks lightly first. A little powder underneath smoothes out the oils and helps your powder blush go on smoother.

- ✔ Gone overboard with blush? Blending a bit of powder over the area tones things down.

- ✔ It's better to build up blush color little by little than to try to correct an overload. If you do get too much color, blend on a little loose powder to tone it down.

- ✔ Brushing a little blush on different areas — lids, brow bone, nose, chin, and forehead — is a quick way to add a little radiance to the face.

- ✔ To boost blush's staying power, or just to give a little more depth to your cheek color, try dusting a bit of powder blush over a cream blush base.

Lip color

I remember watching my mother apply her lipstick. She could do it anywhere, anytime, with or without a mirror, and it always came out perfect. Lip color is one of the quickest and easiest ways to change the look of your face. Not only do you have unlimited colors to choose from, but you can also use all kinds of different application techniques. You can make your lips look fuller, smaller, more balanced, more defined, more *anything* just by changing the way you apply your lip color (see my techniques for working with your specific lip shape in "Shaping lips with color" later in this chapter).

The two basic tools for creating any lip look are lip pencil (also called liner) and lipstick. I use them alone or together, depending on the look I want to achieve. When it comes to lip color, you can really put on your artist's hat; mixing, matching, and getting creative is the key to finding your favorite shades.

Applying lip liner

Here are the two different ways that I apply my lip liner. Hopefully, one of them will work for you.

- ✔ **The dot method:** Draw a dot on each point of the upper lip's bow and then draw two more dots right below them at the bottom of the lower lip (see Figure 14-7). Simply connect the dots and you're done.

- ✔ **The dash method:** Work your way around the edge of the lips by using a series of short, gentle lines that you connect as you go along (see Figure 14-7).

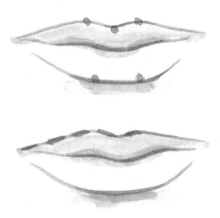

Figure 14-7:
Two easy ways to line the lips: the dot method (top) and the dash method.

Lip liner tipsheet

- ✔ George Newell, one of my favorite makeup artists ever, always started by filling in the corners of my mouth with lip pencil and then lined around the lip. By filling in the corners, he made my lips look fuller and also created a good reference point for applying the rest of the liner.

- ✔ With most lipstick colors, you can use a neutral, lip-toned pencil for lining; but if your lipstick is a vivid or deep shade, use a same-toned pencil to get the most flawless look.

- ✔ Lips filled in with brownish or lip-toned liner look great with lip gloss or lip balm on top.

- ✔ Be sure that your lip pencil is sharpened to a soft point before you begin; if it's too worn down, you'll get a thick, sloppy line.

- ✔ Those chubby lipstick pencils are good for quick color, but their tips are much too broad for careful lining, and their consistency is too creamy to stay put for long. For precise work, go with a classic slim pencil.

- ✔ While lining your lips, don't open your mouth unnaturally wide — you'll distort your natural lip line, making it difficult to see where pencil should be applied.

✔ Lip liner can be applied either before or after other lip color. Use it first to help lipstick adhere better and resist feathering; use it after to help perfect your final lip shape.

Applying lipstick

I use a lip brush when using very dark or vivid shades of lipstick to get a more defined look.

1. **Coat your lip brush evenly with color.**

2. **Beginning at the center of each lip, work your way out toward the mouth's corners.**

   Keep the brush flat against your lip; you'll get cleaner edges and a more even coat of color.

I use lipstick directly from the tube when I'm using colors that don't need precise placement. I put a little across the bottom lip, a little across the top lip, smudge, and I'm usually ready to go. Perfect with a lip pencil if necessary.

I use my fingers for potted gloss or when I just want to stain my lips with color.

Lip color tipsheet

✔ To matte down shine and help color last, blot lips with a tissue and then apply another coat of color. For power-blotting, makeup artist Fran Cooper separates a two-ply tissue, rests one half over the lips, and then dusts on a little loose powder.

✔ For fuller-looking lips, a dab of lip gloss in the center of your finished lips has a glamorous effect. Shinier, prettier textures make lips fuller; matte textures make lips look smaller.

✔ For smoothest application, open your mouth slightly to stretch lips taut. And forget about puckering — it's useless for applying lipstick.

✔ No lip color looks good over dry, chapped lips. Although lipstick's high oil and wax content does help lips stay smooth, lip balm is the better choice — whether alone or under lip color — to keep lips in good shape. If chapping is a perpetual problem, avoid very matte or long-wearing lipsticks, which tend to dry out the lips.

✔ If your lipstick is not going on smoothly because of peeling or chapped lips, use a toothbrush to gently exfoliate.

✔ You don't have to settle for color as it comes out of the tube: Use your lip brush to swirl two or more colors together, use a different lip liner shade as a color-changing base, or layer one shade over another right on your lips.

✔ If you want to wear dark colors without an intense effect, try using a neutral lip pencil to define the shape of the lip, and then apply the color with your fingertip. You'll have to reapply often.

✔ To keep lipstick off your teeth after color's on, stick a finger into your mouth, purse your lips around it, and then draw the finger out. Any extra color comes off on your finger.

Shaping lips with color

Are your lips thinner, fuller, or flatter than you'd like? Here's where you find out how to make the most of what you've got. You already know that lip liner and lipstick are the two must-have tools for creating any kind of redefinition to the lips; you already read about the basic moves in "Applying lip liner" and "Applying lipstick." Now it's time to get a little more personal with specific steps for your specific lip shape.

Hold the line

Tired of lipsticks that give up the ghost as soon as they hit your lips? Try these tricks for making color stay on and stay put:

To Fix This	Do This
Lipstick feathering	Give lips a "base" of foundation or primer before applying color; and/or always use lip liner; and/or lightly powder the lip border to keep color in place; and/or avoid creamy or glossy lip color products.
Lip color fade	Start with a "base" of lip color fixative or foundation; or fill in lips entirely with lip pencil before applying lipstick; or color over lips with pencil after lipstick is applied; and/or apply two to three layers of lip color, blotting well after each; and/or dust lightly with loose powder to set; and/or opt for long-wearing or matte formulas.
Lip gloss loss	Fill in lips with pencil or blotted-down matte lipstick before applying.
Liner "outline"	Fill in both lips entirely with pencil.
Lipstick slide-off	Use a cotton swab to re-edge your lips, or use a sponge wedge to "erase" anything that's gone outside the lines.

Even though the techniques outlined here are corrective in nature, there's still room for fun. Try slight alterations, such as making your upper lip's bow more pointed or rounded; maybe extend your corners slightly for maximum smileage. Just don't get too tricky, and practice until your new lip shape looks like a part of you.

Before you get started, familiarize yourself with Figure 14-8's handy reference to the different parts of the lip. Once you're up to speed, just find your lip type in the following sections and take it from there. Even if you don't have "problem" lips, these principles are still great to know when you want to try something new.

Figure 14-8:
The parts of the lip.

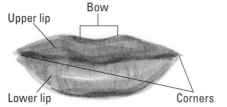

Upper lip • Bow • Lower lip • Corners

Lip type: Thin

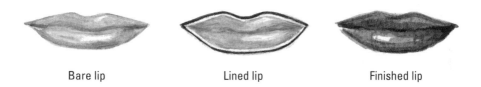

Bare lip   Lined lip   Finished lip

Objective: To maximize lip size by visually enhancing the area

Lip Liner: Line exactly on top of your natural lip line.

Lip Color: Using a lip brush, apply color right up to the outer edge of the liner.

What Works: Glossy finishes add more dimension to lips.

What Doesn't:

- ✔ Matte textures and bright colors look too severe on thin lips.
- ✔ Don't dramatically overdraw the lip line; doing so looks harsh and unnatural, especially up close.

Lip type: Flat

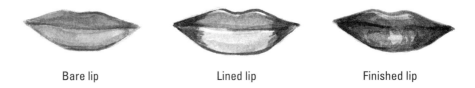

Bare lip   Lined lip   Finished lip

Objective: To create an illusion of greater fullness and projection

Lip Liner: Line lips on top of the natural border and then fill in the corners with pencil.

Lip Color: Apply color, working from the corners inward, fading toward the middle of the lips. Finish with a dab of gloss at lips' center.

What Works:

- ✔ Keeping color at the outer edges of the lips gives the appearance of more depth.
- ✔ Shiny finishes, especially at the center, help round the look of lips.

What Doesn't: Avoid dry, matte textures; their flat finish deflates lips even further.

Lip type: Uneven

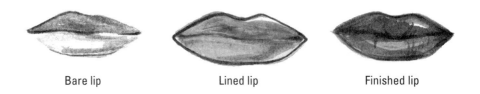

Bare lip   Lined lip   Finished lip

Objective: To equalize out-of-balance lips by redefining their borders

Lip Liner: Line the thinner lip just on top of the natural lip line; line the fuller lip just inside the natural lip line.

Lip Color: Using a lip brush for precision, apply lipstick right to the edge of each line.

What Works: Finishes with subtle sheen help unify the look of the lips.

What Doesn't: Don't try to make the lips perfectly equal; a light reshaping is sufficient.

Lip type: Full

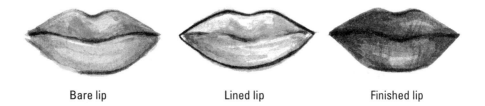

| Bare lip | Lined lip | Finished lip |

Objective: To minimize lip size by visually diminishing the area

Lip Liner: Line lips just inside the natural edge or go without liner.

Lip Color: Use a lip brush to blend color right to the new lip line. Or use your finger just to blend color into the lips.

What Works: Lip-toned lipsticks always look great on full lips.

What Doesn't:

- ✔ Very bright or overly glossy lipsticks only emphasize the dimension of the lips.
- ✔ Gloss all over the lips only makes them look fuller. If you're going to use gloss, use it only in the center.

Lip type: Undefined

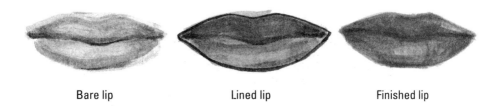

| Bare lip | Lined lip | Finished lip |

Objective: To strengthen lip borders that are faded or uneven

Lip Liner: Draw a dot on each point of the bow and then draw two dots right below on the edge of the lower lip. Working from the corners inward, connect the dots.

Lip Color: Blend color to liner edge with a lip brush.

What Works: Stay with more matte textures to help keep lipstick in place.

What Doesn't: Imprecise application and runny textures blur lip edges even more.

Lip type: Contrasting

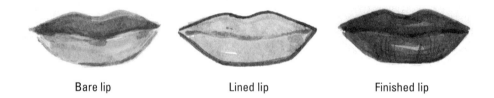

Bare lip   Lined lip   Finished lip

Objective: To equalize the look of different-colored lips

Lip Liner: Cover lips with a light layer of foundation, apply liner at the lip border, and then use liner to fill in lips entirely for longer-lasting color.

Lip Color: Apply lipstick with a brush to avoid removing base color.

What Works: Prep lips to even out the tone before lip color goes on.

What Doesn't:

- ✔ Don't overapply foundation or pencil; too much on the lips makes lips look dry and peely.
- ✔ Some lips are impossible to match exactly, so relax and don't keep redoing.

Lip type: Downturned

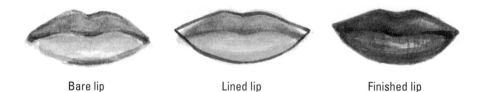

Bare lip   Lined lip   Finished lip

Objective: To redirect the lip line and visually upturn the corners of the mouth

Lip Liner: Start liner on the lower lip, extending the natural line upward at the corners to just above the corner of the upper lip. Line the upper lip, joining it to the point created by the first line. Dust with powder to set.

Lip Color: Smooth on color with a brush, applying very lightly at the corners to avoid lipstick bleed.

What Works: A slight redefinition with pencil brings up the corners.

What Doesn't: Don't attempt to paint on a whole new smile; a slight alteration at the corners is all you're trying to achieve.

Lip type: Mature

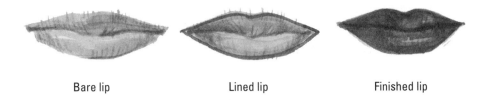

| Bare lip | Lined lip | Finished lip |

Objective: To create stay-put color and prevent lipstick feathering on older lips

Lip Liner: Apply a light base coat of foundation or lip-fix product; gently stretch lips taut between the first two fingers while lining to allow smooth application; lightly powder over liner to set.

Lip Color: Smooth on lipstick with a brush, just to the drawn line; then blot well.

What Works: Create a base with foundation and pencil to give color something to cling to, use powder to help stop lipstick bleed, and look for products with lasting matte textures.

What Doesn't: Avoid overly creamy or glossy textures that slide easily off lips and into fine lines.

Working the Extras

This section talks about a few key makeup items that you may want to pull out from time to time to give your makeup a boost.

Eyelash curler

For some women, this item is not an "extra"; it's a must. If your lashes grow straight (common in Asian women) or turn down at your eye's outer corner, curling the lashes helps give the eye a more open, alert appearance. The most common types of curlers clamp onto the entire top row of lashes; a rarer find is a spot-curler that you can use on specific areas.

Using an eyelash curler

1. **Position the curler on the upper lashes, close to the lash roots.**

   Make sure that the corner lashes are in the curler; they're the most important.

2. **Gently clamp the curler shut, pressing and holding for a few seconds.**

Eyelash curler tipsheet

✔ Lash curling must be done before mascara is applied; otherwise, lashes will stick to the rubber pads and may get pulled out.

✔ Curling lashes is easier if the lid's open only about halfway. Either tilt your head back slightly if you're using a wall mirror, or look downward into a hand-held mirror.

✔ If eye droopiness is a problem and your regular curler doesn't seem to be helping, look for a corner curler. This tool specifically curls the corner lashes that your regular curler might miss, lifting up a droopy eye.

✔ If you notice redness and itching in your eye area, your mascara may not be to blame — you could be allergic to the rubber pads or nickel plating on your eyelash curler. Eliminate curling from your makeup routine and consult a dermatologist if the irritation persists.

Individual eyelashes

If your own lashes are sparse or absent, or you just want to pump up your lash volume for a special occasion, false lashes can't be beat. The only kind of false eyelashes I recommend are the individual lashes. They look the most natural, and you use them only where they're needed.

Applying individual lashes

1. **Curl your own lashes, making sure that the corners are curled up as much as possible.**

2. **Apply mascara.**

3. **Apply a dab of lash adhesive to the back of your hand.**

4. **Using a slant-edge or rounded-tip tweezer, pick up a lash and dip its tip in the glue.**

5. **Begin placing individual lashes from a bit beyond the center mark to the outer corner of the eye, as shown in Figure 14-9. Gently place a lash where desired on top of the eyelid, as close to the lash line as possible.**

6. **Open your eye to check placement and figure out where the next lash is needed.**

   Usually, you need only five to six lashes on each eye.

7. **Apply a second coat of mascara if desired.**

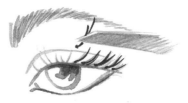

Figure 14-9: Tweezers help you position individual false lashes.

Individual eyelashes tipsheet

- ✔ You can buy many different types of glues. The best ones become transparent when they dry.

- ✔ Individual lashes come in a variety of lengths and thicknesses, so think about the look you're trying to achieve before you buy, and think about what would blend best with your own lash texture and length.

- ✔ Apply false lashes *after* eyeliner is on; liner helps to visually join the lashes to the lid by blurring the line where the lashes meet the lid.

- ✔ Using a magnifying mirror may make applying individual eyelashes easier.

- ✔ To remove individual lashes, remove your eye makeup as usual. When doing so, you'll loosen the glue and you'll slowly be able to lift the lashes away from the lid one by one.

- ✔ Do not re-use individual lashes.

Bronzer

Bronzer is a great way to instantly warm up your face. In the summer, it adds to the tan you may already have, and in the winter, when you're usually paler, it's great for warming up the skin and giving it a healthy glow. Several formulas are available: Choose one that works with your skin, your skill level, and the look you want to create — and be sure to check out some great bronzer effects in the Makeup Workbook color section.

- **Powder** is the quickest and easiest to use and can be found in both loose and pressed form. I use powder bronzer in the winter when less sheen is more appropriate. Powder bronzers without shimmer are usually the best; if you want shimmer, buy a specific shimmer product.

- **Cream** and **stick** bronzers are great for spot placement of color on cheekbones, nose, chin, eyelids, and even lips. They're ideal for the summer months, when more sheen on the skin looks healthy and appropriate. Cream and stick bronzers come in a variety of shades, from pink to peach to brown. Stay away from anything overly orange.

Applying powder bronzer

1. **Apply a small amount of bronzer to your blush brush.**

   Tap off any excess before applying; you'll prevent too-dark or blotchy color.

2. **Begin brushing across your cheeks, forehead, nose, and chin.**

3. **Correct and lighten any overbronzed areas with a clean cotton pad or a little loose powder.**

Applying cream or stick bronzer

1. **Make sure that your skin is clean and moisturized.**

2. **Apply a bit of bronzer to your fingertips; then rub your fingers together so that the bronzer forms a light, even coat.**

3. **Dab the bronzer onto your cheeks and begin to rub it in. For further bronzing, move to your forehead and chin and continue blending. Whatever is left on your fingers can be applied across your nose and eyelids.**

4. **To set, finish with a light dusting of loose powder.**

Bronzer tipsheet

- When using powder bronzer with other makeup formulas like foundation, powder, and blusher, make sure to use your bronzer last, possibly even in place of blusher.

✔ Remember, bronzer is for adding color to the face, not recoloring it altogether. If you're extremely pale, you may have to pass on bronzer. For warming the skin tone, try a loose powder that's one to two shades darker than your natural skin tone.

✔ Bronzer can stain skin if not blended immediately, so work quickly.

✔ If you've used bronzer on your face and are wearing a low-cut dress, you may want to add a little bronzer to key spots on your chest as well.

✔ If you have very oily skin, powder formulas are your best bet; most cream and stick bronzers contain oil.

Shimmer

Shimmer products are wonderful for highlighting specific areas. They look especially alluring in the evening when used on cheeks, eyes, décolletage, and other areas of the body. Depending on the product you're using, there are basically two ways to apply shimmer: with a brush or with your fingers. Either way, make sure to build up and layer the product for more intensity. Hit key areas that need highlighting, such as cheekbones, eyes, décolletage, and shoulders.

Shimmer tipsheet

✔ Remember, shine calls attention to any area where it's placed, so avoid flaws that you'd rather not highlight, such as crepey lids, crow's feet, or rough-textured areas of skin.

✔ Shimmer is really for the evening. If you like a little shimmer during the day, you can buy a blush with a little shimmer in it.

✔ If you've applied shimmer with your fingers, make sure to wash your hands thoroughly afterwards. Shimmer — especially lotion-type formulas — can stain clothes. Make sure to apply shimmer and let it dry before dressing.

✔ If you're using a brush to apply your shimmer, make sure to clean it thoroughly before using it again with my brush-cleaning technique or by dusting it over a tissue until you see no more shimmer.

Checking Your Look

After you complete all your makeup steps, take one last look. Here's a checklist of common slip-ups to look for:

✔ Make sure that you see no line of demarcation between your face and neck.

✔ Check your eyebrows and hair for residual foundation or powder.

✔ Dust off any excess powder.

✔ Remove any concealer that may have ended up on your lower lashes during application.

✔ Make sure that your blush is not streaking or applied too heavily.

✔ Remove any eye shadow sprinkles under the eyes or on the cheeks.

✔ Check lipstick shape up close in a mirror or in a magnifying mirror, and smile to check for lipstick on the teeth.

Now for the final step: *Step back,* literally, and take a look at the overall picture. Chances are you've been about a foot from the mirror the whole time you've been doing your makeup; stepping back lets you view yourself as others will see you, so it's the way to check that everything's in proper balance. If you can, view your makeup in different lights; that way, you'll be sure to look good wherever you go.

Make little alterations, but resist the urge to redo: Overworking your makeup usually only makes things worse. Remember, makeup is an illusion — the overall effect is more important than the tiny details. It's kind of like a painting: Examine it too closely and you lose sight of what the bigger picture's all about.

Chapter 15
Makeup Q & A

· ·

· ·

Ask away! Here are solutions to the most common makeup quandaries.

Trying Something New

Using a new color or trying a new technique can be intimidating, but it's a great way to keep your look fresh. This section tackles a couple of questions about being adventurous with your makeup.

I really want to change my look. How should I go about it?

Take small steps. Start by playing with the makeup you already own to create different effects (check out Chapter 19 for ideas). Try adding a new lipstick or eye shadow color to your repertoire, or replacing a makeup product that you've been wearing for years with a newer formula. Have a makeup artist or makeup-maven friend help you reassess your look and suggest new directions. Check out magazines and movies for inspiration on new looks or products to try. And see "Getting Out of a Rut" in Chapter 11.

I really want to try a bold new color, but I'm a little hesitant. What's the best way to start?

One eye-catching shade is sufficient for any face, so pick your target — eyes or lips — and work your way into it gradually:

- ✔ With a bright eye shadow shade, try blending it very lightly over your lid until it leaves just a sheer impression of color. You can also mix it with loose powder or a neutral shadow to "dilute" the shade, or use it sparingly near your lash line to give your eyeliner a new effect.

- ✔ On lips, ease into a bold new lipstick by sheering it down with petroleum jelly or lip gloss. Also, try mixing the shade with neutrals that you already own to take off the edge, or blot it down to just a sheer stain of color.

Once you feel comfortable with the look of the new color on your face, you can up the intensity a bit more. Remember, though, that a very bold shade draws attention to *itself,* sometimes taking the focus away from the entirety of your face, so use restraint.

Doing Your Makeup for Special Situations

Whether your "special situation" is as big as a wedding or as small as a weekend trip to a hot climate, you may have questions about how to change your makeup accordingly. This section addresses many of the situations that you may face.

My 13-year-old daughter wants to start wearing makeup. How should I start her off?

The most common mistake that makeup novices make is piling on the product, so concentrate on fun accent items that are difficult to overdo: lip gloss, mascara, and maybe a sheer powder blush. Go together to buy her first products: That way, you won't be surprised to see what she's wearing, and she won't feel dictated-to. Keep in mind that she will, at times, come home with bright, gaudy shades and glittery textures. It's just a phase. We all wore some pretty hideous things in our day, so try to grin and bear it.

As she matures into her later teens, she'll want to add more products to her repertoire. Young skin rarely needs the coverage of foundation, but an oil-free tinted moisturizer can help even out her skin if breakouts are a problem. She can also use concealer or pressed powder to help hide blemishes and control shine. Eyeliner and eye shadow are favorites for experimentation. Your biggest challenge is to convince her that less is more. A fully made-up, matte-powdered face is way too much for a teen; help her satisfy her urge for *more* by encouraging her to try new colors as opposed to overapplying those she has.

Most girls become interested in tweezing their eyebrows as they reach their later teens. Your guidance here is very important; you'll both find it helpful to review the section on brow-shaping in Chapter 13. Start her off with the most basic cleanup and let her maintain what you've done when regrowth occurs. If she really wants to change the shape of her brow, help her do so — slowly — over a period of weeks, supervising all the way. Other good options:

✓ Using brow-grooming gels to give the area a more finished appearance

✓ Enhancing brows with color instead of tweezing

✓ Going to a professional for shapings

What's the best way to do my makeup for a job interview?

Even if you're seeking a job in a "creative" profession (advertising, fashion, and so on), you want to project a polished and professional image when meeting a prospective employer. Keep your makeup understated: You want the interviewer to focus on your qualifications — not your flaming fuchsia lips. Go with muted, natural colors and pay close attention to the grooming aspect of makeup: Foundation and blush should be well-blended; eyes well-defined and smudge-free; lipstick on lips, not teeth. Take a pressed-powder compact with you for last-minute shine control. And remember to make eye contact and smile. (For more help with interview protocol, see Joyce Lain Kennedy's *Job Interviews For Dummies,* also published by IDG Books Worldwide, Inc.)

How do I change my makeup for photography, TV, or video?

If you'll be outdoors, you don't need a lot of adjustment: Just check your look in daylight and make sure that your face is well-powdered to keep shine under control. Indoors is another story: Bright lights tend to drain color from your face and accentuate every little flaw, so you need to make a few changes to your normal routine:

- ✔ Give your skin an even tone and texture by using both foundation and concealer. Apply both with a slightly heavier hand than you normally would; you need the extra coverage under such tight scrutiny.

- ✔ Apply a very light dusting of bronzer to pale skin to help "warm up" the tone. If you'll be in front of the camera regularly, compensate for lighting's wash-out effect by investing in foundation and powder a shade deeper than you normally wear.

- ✔ Powder, powder, powder! Glaring lights intensify shine, so although your skin may look too matte for real life, it will be fine on camera. Avoid shiny finishes, too — glossy lips, sparkly shadows.

- ✔ Don't overdo the eye makeup. Brows need to be well-defined, so fill them in if necessary and groom them into place. Even out lid color with light, neutral shades and keep liner soft. Finish lashes with a few coats of mascara, combing well to declump.

- ✔ Intensify your blusher application and go for lipstick in medium-bright shades. You'll need the extra oomph because bright lights tend to "blow out" color from the face.

- ✔ Keep everything precisely applied: lipstick held in place with lip liner, eyeliner set with powder or shadow, and blush right *on* cheeks, not below. Sloppy application looks even sloppier when magnified by a camera lens, so don't rush.

I'm getting married soon. What should I do about my makeup for the ceremony?

You may want to wow the groom with a great new look on your wedding day, but I must warn you against it. Not only will he be wondering who the stranger is under the veil, but *you'll* be wondering what you were thinking when you look at your wedding photos five years later. The best makeup for your Big Day lets you look like *you* — granted, a you who looks exquisitely put-together with the help of well-chosen makeup.

Consider enlisting the help of a makeup artist for your wedding day. Make sure to have a "dress rehearsal" a few weeks before the wedding so you know that the makeup artist you chose can create a look you love. Another option if you feel confident in your application skills: Have a consultant give you a makeup lesson that teaches you to do it yourself. Some department-store makeup counters, salons, and makeup boutiques also do bridal makeup consultations; contact your local favorite to see whether it offers such services.

If you're doing your makeup yourself, a no-fail approach is to stay with gentle, neutral tones (see the Makeup Workbook color section for ideas). You should already have all your makeup basics together (reread this section if you don't); from there you just need to make a few adjustments:

- ✔ If you're wearing a white dress, wear white while practicing your makeup. Color seems more intense when worn against white, so seeing the contrast helps you adjust your application.

- ✔ Adjust your makeup for the time of day. If you're having an outdoor wedding at noon, use a lighter hand and check your makeup in full daylight; for an evening candlelight wedding, you need to add more intensity to compensate for low light.

- ✔ Define your eyes softly and finish with a couple of well-combed coats of waterproof mascara.

- ✔ Avoid anything that shimmers or sparkles anywhere on the face, including iridescent eye shadow and heavy lip gloss. They'll create a glaring reflection in every flash photo.

- ✔ Apply slightly more blush than normal, still making sure that it's well blended, because photo flash and video lights can make you look washed-out.

- ✔ Keep lips soft and natural-looking, defined with a neutral pencil and filled in with a neutral shade.

- ✔ Have a bridesmaid carry powder, lipstick, and a mirror for you on your wedding day so that you can touch up whenever necessary. Doing so may be a little bothersome, but seeing 100 pictures of yourself when you're not looking your best is worse.

I wear glasses. Do I have to adjust my eye makeup?

Maybe. If your glasses are very thick, you need to be aware of how your lenses distort the look of your eye. Lenses to correct nearsightedness make the eye seem to recede; if you're going for a dramatic eye look, you have to intensify your liner and eye shadow to compensate. Corrective lenses for farsightedness magnify the eyes, so less intensity keeps the eyes from looking even more prominent.

If you're still wearing very thick lenses, ask your ophthalmologist about the newer types of eyeglass lenses. Far thinner and lighter than the old standard, these new lenses practically eliminate the eye distortion and nose-denting weight that are common in strong-prescription lenses. (Contact lenses are also much more advanced now — even if you've had problems in the past, you should be able to find some that are right for you.)

As far as frames go, no one pays attention to those shape-and-color rules anymore. Try on anything that you find attractive, and go with whatever makes you feel good. Do keep *one* key point in mind: A high bridge adds the illusion of length to the nose, and a low bridge visually shortens the nose. And remember, whenever you take your glasses off, check to see that your foundation hasn't piled up where they were resting on your face.

Do I need to change my makeup according to the climate I'm in?

Yes, especially if you're in extreme environmental conditions.

- ✔ Very dry, arid climates (which can be cold, snowy areas as well as the desert) can quickly deplete the skin's moisture; you want to protect your face with a hydrating, protective foundation formula to help your skin stay supple, and perhaps even add a moisturizer underneath.

- ✔ In a very hot, humid climate, you may have trouble literally keeping makeup on your skin. Pare down your application — applying a full face of makeup that you'll only sweat off is a losing battle — and opt for lightweight, water-resistant or waterproof formulas.

- ✔ If you live in a temperate region that has distinct hot and cold seasonal cycles, you know that what works in January is definitely not right for July. Adjust your makeup to accommodate changes throughout the year.

Troubleshooting Makeup Emergencies

Even when you try to do everything right, some days you may end up with a bad case of Wrong. It's inevitable — but not irreversible. This section walks you through some common makeup disasters and tells you how to fix them.

My skin is oily, and my makeup seems to change color a couple hours after I apply it. Why is this happening?

The color change in your makeup is due to the oil that your skin produces. It can seep into color products like blush, making them look shades darker on your skin, and give your foundation and powder an unflattering, orangey tone. The solution: Use oil-free products that are formulated to stand up to oily skin without discoloring. Most contain added oil-absorbing ingredients (such as kaolin) to help the color stay true throughout the day.

Whenever I wear a very deep lip color, it stains my skin. What's the best way to remove it?

Staining often happens when you wear heavily pigmented shades or you wear the same vivid color every day. Try giving your lips a base coat of foundation, neutral-toned lip pencil, or a lipstick fixative product before applying your lipstick. At night, remove every trace of color with makeup remover; if color remains, gently exfoliate your lips with your toothbrush to help loosen set-in pigment. You should also give your lips a rest from the same color every day: Try mixing up your color selection and wearing only lip balm or a light gloss when you're at home.

What's the best way to wake up tired eyes?

First, soothe your eyes with cool compresses or cooling eye gel to help them physically feel more alert and take down the swelling. Use eyedrops for moisture and to reduce redness. Then keep your makeup simple: Even out lid color with foundation or concealer, and then sweep on a light, neutral-toned shadow to help open up the area. Avoid deep shades of eye shadow and liner; they mimic the tones of undereye circles, making them more noticeable. Apply concealer where needed under the eye and all the way to the hollow beside the nose (an old trick for brightening the area). Finish with a good brow brush-up and a couple natural-looking coats of mascara.

My lashes are very short and thin. What can I do?

If your lashes are long enough, use an eyelash curler to help them turn upward, which creates an illusion of more length (particularly if your lashes grow straight). Be sure to let mascara dry between coats so that the next one has something to adhere to. (Remember, some mascaras are better at lengthening, some are better at volumizing, and some can do both, so look around until you find a formula you like.) Place deep, smoky eyeliner near the lash line to give an impression of thicker lashes. If you're still not satisfied, you may want to check into individual (false) eyelashes. Chapter 14 discusses the different types and tells you how to use them.

My eyebrows and lashes have fallen out from chemotherapy. What can I do?

You can approximate your absent brows and lashes with subtly applied makeup. A brow pencil is perfect for redrawing where hairs no longer exist; see the step-by-step instructions in Chapter 14. To simulate the look of lashes, smudge a deep-toned eyeliner right where your lash line would be. On the rest of the eye, stay subtle.

Even though your eye area is your main concern, you may also be looking pale and sallow as a result of your treatment. Foundation helps even out your skin tone, while soft shades of blush and lipstick are great for bringing color to your face. For more beauty advice specific to chemotherapy patients' needs, contact Look Good, Feel Better at 800-395-LOOK (404-329-5763 for international readers), on the Web at www.lgfb.org, or through your local American Cancer Society office. And don't worry — everything should grow back normally once your course of chemo is complete.

I'm having a Bad Skin Day. Help!

I've had my fair share of skin problems, so I know all about Bad Skin Days. You're breaking out, you don't know what to do, and all you really want to do is hide. But I learned that you should *not* try to cover everything with a thick coat of foundation: Trust me, the more you put on, the worse it looks. The best thing you can do is to try to get a little of the redness out of your skin so that you feel more comfortable.

Very sparingly, dot on foundation where you need it, and cover it lightly with powder. After your skin looks a little more even, concentrate on drawing attention to other parts of your face. Maybe go a little deeper with your eye makeup, or give yourself a glossy, natural mouth. Stay away from red lipstick, though — it brings out the redness in your skin.

I have acne-scarred skin and enlarged pores. What's the best way to even out the texture of my face?

Acne scars and pores are less noticeable when your skin doesn't show shine. First, apply a light coat of foundation to help even out your skin tone and texture (use an oil-free formula if your skin is still actively oily). Don't try to fill in recessed scars with extra product: You'll get a heavy, cakey effect that won't improve things in the least. Finish by pressing loose powder evenly onto the face with a puff — you'll give your skin a very smooth, matte appearance that takes attention away from imperfections.

What can I do to cover my freckles?

If you have just a few light freckles on your nose or cheeks, a little foundation helps even things out. Heavily freckled skin, however, is another story. Covering unwanted freckles with a thick coat of foundation may make them disappear — but also makes you look like you're wearing a (none-too-pretty) mask. Instead of trying to hide your natural pigmentation, sparingly blend on a lightweight foundation or tinted moisturizer to help your skin look a bit more polished — or forego foundation altogether and just use powder and concealer where needed.

I have dark skin, and no matter how well I blend my foundation, it looks ashy. What's wrong?

Your foundation probably contains too much talc or titanium dioxide. These ingredients can leave a pasty appearance on dark skin that no amount of blending can rectify. Check labels so that you avoid these ingredients, and remember, when you're buying foundation, you *must* try it on your face to be sure that you're getting the best match and the most flattering finish. See the foundation-buying guidelines in Chapter 11.

I made a mistake when applying my makeup. How do I fix it?

Oops! Whether your hand slipped, you got carried away, or you just went too far, you can always fix these makeup mistakes without going back to the drawing board:

- ✔ **Too-heavy foundation:** You have several options here:
    - Spray your face with a very fine mist of water and blot with a tissue.
    - Blend with a damp makeup sponge.
    - Dab a little moisturizer on your fingers and blend over your face.
- ✔ **Overpowdered face:** Try any of these tricks:
    - Whisk away excess powder with a powder brush.
    - Press the powder into your face with a velvet puff.
    - Lightly spray the face with a fine mist of water.
- ✔ **Cakey concealer:** Dab a little moisturizer onto the area and blend.
- ✔ **Overcolored eyebrows:** Brush in a little loose powder, or use a hard toothbrush lightly coated with a neutral eye shadow and comb upward.
- ✔ **Too-dark eye shadow:** Blend loose powder over the lid.
- ✔ **Hard-looking eyeliner:** Either cover the line with loose powder or a lighter-toned eye shadow, or blend over the area with a brush or sponge-tip applicator (dry or damp).
- ✔ **Clumpy eyelashes:** Use a lash comb to remove clumps.
- ✔ **Mascara smudge:** Dampen a cotton swab with water or non-oily eye makeup remover, press onto the smudge with a blotting or twisting motion, and spot-reapply makeup if necessary.
- ✔ **Too much blush:** Blend loose powder over blush, or use a cotton ball to pick up a bit of color.
- ✔ **Too-bright lipstick:** Blot and then blend on a deeper or more neutral shade.
- ✔ **Too-dark lipstick:** Blot and then top-coat with a lighter shade, or blot it down to a stain, putting lip gloss or lip balm on top to make it look moist and natural. You can also use a dot of foundation mixed with lip gloss to lighten the color.
- ✔ **Lopsided lipstick:** Clean up anything over the lip line with a sponge wedge or cotton swab (dipped in makeup remover if the color is dense). Reapply foundation, if needed, with the edge of a sponge; then redefine the lip border with a lip pencil or brush.
- ✔ **Too-dry lipstick:** Add a coat of lip balm or gloss.

How do I deal with adverse reactions to makeup products?

If your skin is at all sensitive or allergic, or if you're trying to avoid potential problems, check your makeup products for the ingredients listed in Table 15-1. These are just the tip of the iceberg; hundreds of different ingredients are known to cause allergic reactions, so the ones that bother you may not be named here. Anytime you have an adverse reaction to *anything,* stop using the product immediately. If the irritation doesn't improve within 48 hours, consult a dermatologist.

Table 15-1	Common Cosmetic Irritants
Ingredient	*Used In*
Alcohol, SD alcohol	Some foundations
*Fragrance	Every type of cosmetic
Glycols (including glycerin and propylene glycol)	Foundation, mascara, lip color
Lanolin and derivatives	Every type of cosmetic
Mica	Powder shadows and blushes
Mineral oil and petrolatum	Every type of cosmetic
*Preservatives	Every type of cosmetic; common culprits include imidazolidinyl urea; Quaternium 1-15; parabens (methyl-, propyl-, butyl-, ethyl-); DHA, BHT, BHA and EDTAs

* Known to be the most irritating ingredients used in cosmetics

What can I do when I forget a makeup product at home or am running out of a product?

You're out of town for a friend's wedding when it dawns on you: Your makeup bag is back at home, perched nicely on the edge of the bathroom sink. Or when you're in a panic to get out the door, you suddenly find a foundation bottle full of nothing. Luckily for you, Table 15-2 lists some makeup products that do a pretty good job of pinch-hitting for one another, and also lists some tricks that stretch your makeup before it's completely gone.

Table 15-2	Making the Most of Your Makeup Products	
Product	**To Replace It**	**To Stretch It**
Liquid foundation	Pressed or loose powder	Add water or very thin moisturizer a few drops at a time; shake well. (**Note:** If you do add water to a product, boil the water first and let it cool before using it — you don't want to introduce any germs into the product.)
Concealer	Two layers of foundation	
Pressed powder	Facial tissue or blotting papers (see Chapter 12)	Remove what's left in the pan and crush with a spoon; apply with a powder brush (or mix in with your loose powder).
Loose powder	Pressed powder applied with a brush	Mix with baby powder.
Blush	Lipstick	Dig the remainder out of the pan and crush to a powder with the underside of a spoon. Store in a small container and/or mix with a little petroleum jelly to recycle as glossy, new lip colors. (Also works for powder eye shadow.)
Eyeliner	Wet eye shadow	
Lip liner	Neutral eye pencil	
Lipstick	Blush mixed with lip balm	Dig the product out of the tube with a toothpick; store in a small, airtight container and apply with a brush.

How can I keep my makeup looking perfect all day long?

Start by using makeup formulas that are right for your skin. If your skin is very oily, for example, oil-based products slide right off your face. Review Chapter 11 to figure out which products work best for you.

The real key to keeping things in place is powder, which comes into play in two ways. Because liquid and cream formulas tend to travel when body heat warms them, powder-form color (blush and eye shadow) is a longer-lasting option. No matter what formulas you choose, use loose powder to set your makeup after it's on: Not only does it "seal" foundation and concealer, but you can also apply it to your eyes and lips to keep liner and lipstick in place.

Part IV
Home Spa

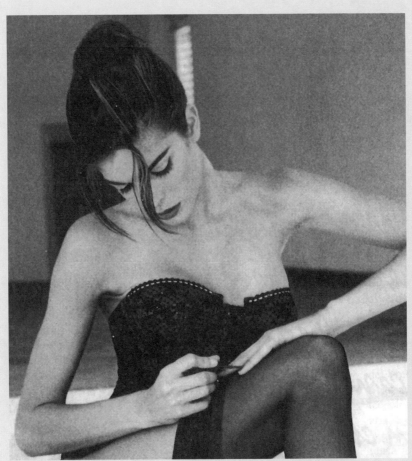

In this part . . .

Regular grooming and pampering not only makes you feel better about yourself but also is a necessity to keep your appearance at its best. Every month or so, give yourself the gift of a home spa. Dedicate an hour or two to total self-indulgence, and you'll be amazed at how much better your look and feel. This part gives you my personal tips for setting up a spa in your very own bathroom.

Chapter 16
Stephanie's Home Spa Regimen

· ·

In This Chapter

▶ Saving time, money, and your sanity with a home spa night

▶ Purchasing the ingredients you need

▶ Pampering your hair, face, and body

▶ Step-by-step instructions for home manicures and pedicures

· ·

*L*ike many women, I often get busy with my kids or work and forget to do the little things to keep myself looking my best. So once a month, I like to take a little time for myself and turn my bathroom into my personal spa. In this chapter, I give you my recipe for a relaxing spa night.

What You Need

My home spa night (and I *always* do it at night) includes a deep hair-conditioning treatment, hair removal for face and body, exfoliation of face and body skin, a facial, and a manicure and pedicure. Before you can get started, you need a few things stored away in your bathroom. I normally keep these things in my bathroom cabinet at all times so that whenever I find the time or feel that I need to turn my bathroom into a home spa, it's easy and the products are readily available. Following is a list of the products you need to turn your own bathroom into a home spa. All these items are for either grooming or relaxation.

✔ Candles (scented candles are especially soothing)

✔ Deep-conditioning treatment for your hair

✔ Shower cap

✔ Facial cleanser

- Facial mask for your skin type (see Chapter 2)
- Eyebrow tweezers
- Cream hair bleach
- Cream hair remover
- Lavender bath salts or essential oils for the bath
- Loofah
- Epsom salts
- Orangewood stick
- Pumice stone
- Cool cloth or sliced cucumbers (to rest over your eyes)
- Thick body moisturizer (such as cocoa butter moisturizer)
- Eye cream
- Light facial moisturizer
- Lip balm

TIP

Aromatherapy

Aromatherapy is a word that was first used in the field of massage therapy to describe massages given with essential oils, which are distilled herb and plant essences. Today, the term *aromatherapy* encompasses all treatments and products that use the scents of herbs, flowers, fruits, and other plants that are known to have therapeutic properties.

Thanks to aromatherapy's popularity, many products are now available for use in home spas. Using aromatherapy in your home can be as simple as infusing fresh or dried herbs in your bath, adding a few drops of essential oil to bowls of water in the bathroom, or lighting a scented candle.

Here are some of the plants and herbs that have been used for healing, purification, and cleansing throughout the centuries:

- **Relaxing/calming:** Lavender, rose, geranium, marjoram, sandalwood, chamomile, lemongrass, lemon balm, palmarosa

- **Uplifting:** Ylang-Ylang, clary sage, bergamot, tangerine, geranium, coriander, cypress, grapefruit, orange, sage, tea tree, thyme

- **Invigorating/stimulating:** Rosemary, mint, ginger, basil, camphor, lemon, wintergreen, bay, birch, cardamom, nutmeg, pine, juniper

The Ritual

Pick a time when you can be alone for an hour and a half. For me, that's usually after I put my three boys to bed. I start by getting myself a big glass of water with lemon. The heat of the bath always makes me thirsty, and after all, any great spa has plenty of water with lemon on hand. To create a relaxing environment in my bathroom, I light some candles and may even listen to relaxing music. Of course, I keep all the lights on when tweezing my eyebrows or doing anything that requires light. Once you're ready to soak in the tub, you can turn the lights out.

I begin by deep-conditioning my hair. (See Chapter 5 for more information about deep conditioners.) I dampen my hair, put the conditioner in, coat the ends thoroughly, wrap it up in a shower cap to hold in moisture, and then wrap a towel around that to keep the conditioner off my skin. Then I wash my face and use an exfoliating mask, and then, depending on what my skin needs, I may apply one other mask. Use the mask that best suits your skin at that time, whether it's moisturizing or drying for oilier skin types. When my skin is unbalanced or irritated, I may use organic yogurt as a mask — it soothes the skin and brings the pH balance back in balance. Apply a thick layer all over the face, leave it on for five minutes, and then rinse with cool water.

Next, I tweeze my eyebrows, check for any other unwanted hairs on the face, and trim or pluck if necessary. I also bleach any hairs on my face or body that are darker than I want them to be. Or if the hair on my face is too abundant to bleach, I use a cream hair remover, because waxing causes my face to break out.

If I haven't had a manicure or pedicure recently, I file my nails and brush and clean them. But I wait until I'm submerged in the bath to push back my cuticles. The warm water makes the cuticles easier to push back, and it gives you a little something to do so that you don't get bored while soaking in the tub. Obviously, if you're going to polish your fingernails and toenails, do so *after* the bath. The section "Caring for Your Hands and Feet," later in this chapter, gives the instructions for a professional-looking home manicure and pedicure.

Now it's time to prep the bath and add some bath salts or a few drops of essential oil. Lavender bath salts are my absolute favorite. The scent is reviving and soothing at the same time.

I use a loofah and handfuls of Epsom salts directly on dampened skin to exfoliate the skin on my body. Epsom salts are wonderful — not only are they inexpensive (you can buy a half-gallon jug at a grocery store for a couple of dollars) — but they're also great for soaking your muscles and exfoliating the skin on your body. Don't use Epsom salts if you're going to shave your legs. Either shave the next day or just loofah to exfoliate. Epsom salts can irritate freshly shaven legs.

Home remedies

Yogurt isn't the only food that comes in handy as a beauty basic. I use ingredients such as honey and baby oil combined on my body to make my skin incredibly soft (just make sure to rinse it off before you get out of the bath); shredded cucumbers packed onto my face to relieve puffiness; or milk to rinse my face and add a smooth, balanced texture to the skin. These are some fun recipes to try at home as long as you don't mind cleaning up the mess. I don't recommend using food products in your hair, though. Eggs and oils are just too difficult to rinse out completely.

Now it's time to push back the cuticles on my hands and feet. I keep it simple by using an orangewood stick or my thumbnail. I also rub my feet with a pumice stone to smooth the calluses. Then I lie back and rest with a cool cloth or cucumber slices on my eyes until I'm ready to get out of the tub. Remember to try to soak for a good 20 minutes to get the full impact of the essentials oils or bath salts on your skin and muscles.

After I finish soaking, I thoroughly rinse the deep conditioner out of my hair. I towel-dry my hair and let it air-dry to give it a break from styling. For the finishing touch, I usually take advantage of spa night to put on a thick moisturizer, such as a cocoa butter moisturizer; then I put on my bathrobe and let it soak in. Eye cream, a light moisturizer, and a little lip balm are the last steps unless I'm in the mood to paint my nails. Remember, if you're going to polish your nails, they must be free of all oils for the best results.

Caring for Your Hands and Feet

Elisa Ferri, who has written several books on manicures and pedicures, is also well-known in the fashion industry for giving models clean, modern-looking hands and feet. In this section, Elisa gives her personal regimen for great-looking nails. Here's what you need:

- 100 percent pure cotton balls
- Moisturizing nail polish remover
- Two different grades of emery boards: one coarse, one fine
- An orangewood stick to push back cuticles and clean under nails (never a metal pusher)

✔ Cuticle softener

✔ Cuticle nipper

✔ Bowl of warm, sudsy water

✔ Moisturizer or nail oil

✔ Foot scraper or a pumice stone

Manicure

Follow these steps for a perfect manicure:

1. **Remove any old polish.**

   Place a cotton pad or ball on the nail for a moment and then swipe outward to prevent smearing. Repeat as necessary. Make sure that you're using a nail polish remover that has a conditioning agent, which is less drying.

2. **File the nails.**

   Nails come in many shapes, from the classic oval to a soft square. If you have a very narrow nail bed, you don't want your nails to be too oval or pointed — a soft square is better. If you have a particularly wide nail base, you can narrow it down a bit by making the nail more oval. You may need to experiment to find the right shape for you.

   Using a smooth, soft emery board, file back and forth, being careful not to file deep into the nail corners, which can make the nail fragile. (See Figure 16-1.)

   Remember the old adage that said never to file back and forth? Although that was good advice in the days of metal nail files, it really doesn't hold true today, as long as you use a fairly soft emery board.

3. **Push back the cuticles and clean the nails.**

   Put a cuticle softener on the cuticle edges and then place your hands in warm, soapy water. The water loosens up any dirt that may be underneath your nails, making it easy to remove, and softens the cuticles so that they can be pushed back. If you've been working in the garden and you have stubborn dirt underneath your nails, use a soft nail brush or toothbrush to scrub over and under your nails.

   After you soak, you can clean underneath the free edge of your nails with an orangewood stick — never use anything metal. Push back the cuticles by using either a soft towel (as shown in Figure 16-2) or an orangewood stick wrapped in cotton. If you have a hangnail, trim it with a cuticle nipper.

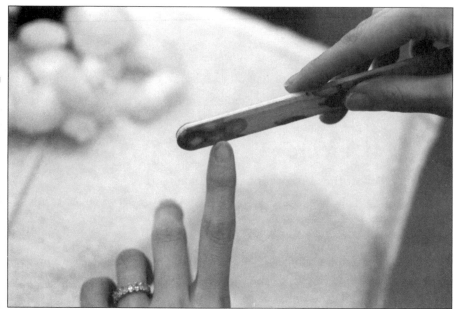

Figure 16-1:
File your nails gently back and forth. If your nail beds are narrow, a soft square is better; if they are wide, make the nails more oval.

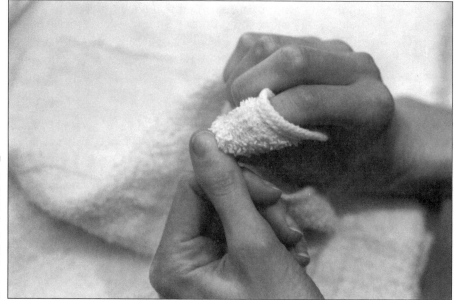

Figure 16-2:
Wrap a soft towel around your fingertip to push back your cuticles.

Never let a manicurist cut your cuticles. Cuticle cutting was just an unnecessary fad. Removing the cuticle takes away the nail's protective barrier, which prevents foreign particles such as food and bacteria from getting underneath the skin.

4. **Massage the nails.**

   Massage with hand cream, and be generous. Using your thumbs, work in a circular motion. Then take a cotton-wrapped orangewood stick dipped in nail polish remover and swipe thoroughly over each nail to remove any creamy residue, leaving a clean surface to which you can apply your polish.

5. **Buff or polish the nails.**

   You can now either polish your nails or leave them clean. If you choose to leave them clean, take a buffer and gently work all over the nail surface in a side-to-side motion. Then take a moisturizer or nail oil and work it into and around the entire nail, including the cuticle. Doing so prevents breakage, splitting, and damage due to dryness. If you want to polish, follow these steps:

   1. **Apply a base coat.**

      A base coat smoothes the nail surface and helps the polish adhere better and last longer. Only one coat is necessary.

   2. **Apply polish.**

      Make sure that the polish is mixed well; then apply in quick, light strokes. Dip the brush into the polish only once. Make your first stroke at the center of the nail and follow it with one sweep along each side, as shown in Figure 16-3. This technique helps prevent excess polish on the nail edges. Apply two coats.

   3. **Remove the excess polish.**

      Dip an orangewood stick into polish remover and then gently swipe around the edges of the nail and the free edge.

   4. **Apply a top coat.**

      The top coat adds protection and enhances the polish's shine. One coat is sufficient; apply as in Step 2.

   5. **To extend the life of the manicure, add one new coat of clear polish every day.**

For polishing, a base coat, a polish, and a top coat combined give the most professional look and last the longest.

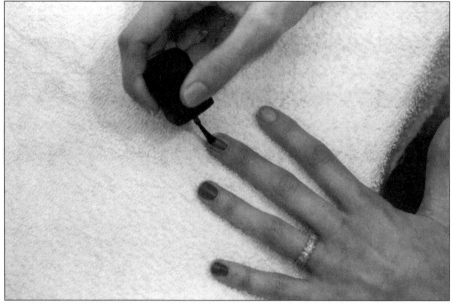

Figure 16-3:
Apply one stroke of polish down the middle of the nail, and then follow with one sweep down each side.

Pedicure

A perfect pedicure includes trimming, shaping, and polishing toenails, as well as removing dead skin and softening calluses. Follow these steps:

1. **Remove any existing polish.**

2. **Clip and file the nails straight across.**

   Always keep toenails short and straight across. If you file in a round shape into the corners, you're likely to get ingrown toenails.

3. **If you're going to do just a toenail polish change, use a rough emery board to slough off dead skin and calluses. Rinse off the dust and moisturize; then skip down to Step 9.**

4. **Apply cuticle softener around your cuticles and then soak your feet in a soapy bath for five to ten minutes.**

   You can add Epsom salts to the water to relieve sore muscles in your feet.

5. **Use a foot file or pumice stone on the bottoms of your feet and toes or wherever you find dry skin or callus growths.**

   Be careful not to file too much, or you may cause irritation. If you use a pumice stone, rub in a circular motion.

6. **Push back your cuticles with an orangewood stick or a towel wrapped around your thumb. Clean the dirt from underneath your toenails with the other end of the orangewood stick.**

   If you have a painful hangnail, trim it. Otherwise, leave your cuticles alone.

7. **Remove your feet from the bath and dry them with a towel, making sure to dry between your toes.**

8. **Apply moisturizing lotion all over your feet.**

   For an invigorating foot massage, rub your feet with peppermint foot lotion, working your thumbs in a circular motion.

9. **Insert toe separators or folded tissues between your toes, as shown in Figure 16-4.**

10. **Using an orangewood stick wrapped in cotton and soaked in nail polish remover, swipe the toenails and nail edges until clean.**

11. **Apply a base coat, two coats of color, and a top coat.**

    Follow the same instructions for applying polish to your fingernails. Let the polish dry for one minute between coats.

I suggest polishing your toes close to bedtime and putting on the top coat the following morning so that you give your toenails enough time to dry without getting sheet marks. Also, after ten minutes, put your thumb over a bottle of olive or baby oil and rub it over the top of your toenails. Doing so helps prevent them from smudging and also moisturizes your cuticles.

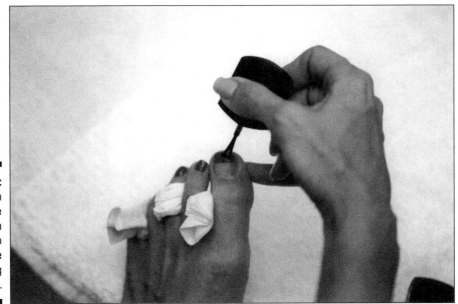

Figure 16-4:
You can place tissue between your toes to make polishing easier.

The benefits of steam

If you have access to a steam room through a spa, at a gym, or in your own home, remember that steam is great for your skin and also reduces stress. A steam room is a nice place to throw a little deep conditioner in your hair and sit for a while. Just be sure to drink lots of water during or after your steam to rehydrate your body.

Part V
The Part of Tens

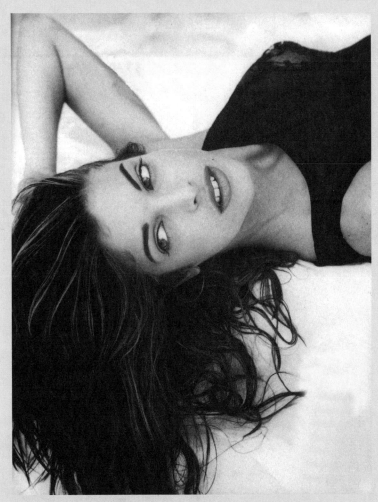

Patrick Demarchelier

In this part . . .

*E*very *...For Dummies* book has a Part of Tens, full of quick tips and helpful advice. In this part, I list some great products that you can purchase at drugstores, beauty supply stores, and salons without spending a fortune. I also give you ideas for varying your makeup look without having to buy any new products. So whether you're in the mood to shop or just stay home and experiment with your makeup, this part is full of useful tips and tricks that can help you.

Chapter 17

Ten Terrific Items to Pick Up at a Drugstore

In This Chapter
▶ Great finds at the corner drugstore
▶ Products that don't cost a fortune but still work great

Many women think that to get quality, you have to spend a lot of money. But in many cases, that just isn't true. In this chapter, I list several products that I use myself that you can pick up for very little cost at almost any drugstore.

Aussie Miracle Shampoo and Conditioner

Aussie Miracle shampoo and conditioner are great for all hair types and for natural or chemically treated hair. The "Miracle" part is the deep conditioning and moisturizing that these products do.

Bonne Bell Lip Smacker

To keep my lips from chapping, I wear some sort of lip balm at all times. Bonne Bell Lip Smacker has been one of my favorite products since I was a teenager. It hydrates the lips, adds sheen, tastes great, and comes in a variety of flavors, all with their own unique hint of color.

Caress Body Wash

Regular soap can be drying to the skin. Try Caress body wash instead — it moisturizes as it cleanses, is gentle on the skin, smells fresh, and comes in a bottle for easy use in the shower. It also works well as a shaving lotion for your legs.

Cetaphil Facial Cleanser

This classic skin care product is great for all skin types. Because it cleans without irritating the skin or stripping away natural oils, many doctors recommend it.

Clearasil Tinted Cream

This acne medication, when used moderately, can help dry up the occasional pimple. (If you use too much or use it too often, you'll dry out your skin, because it contains benzoyl peroxide, a drying ingredient.) You can find out more about this popular product at the Clearasil Web site, www.clearasil.com.

Cotton Rounds

One hundred percent cotton rounds are better than cotton balls. You can use them to remove cosmetics, nail polish, and mascara; apply astringent; and, when wet, to remove cleanser. My favorite brand is Swispers.

Cream or Powder Blusher

Most brands of blush are comparable, so this is a great product to save a bit of money on. Revlon makes my favorite blush; it's the one for mature skin. Shopping at the drugstore is a great way to find a new shade or add to your existing makeup collection without spending a fortune.

Epsom Salts

Epsom salts are wonderful for exfoliating dead skin cells and giving the skin a fresh, healthy glow; I use them in the bath or shower whenever I do a home spa night (see Chapter 16 for details).

Humidifier

If you have problems with dry skin that you can't seem to remedy, try a humidifier — it will probably solve your problem. Humidifiers are great during the winter or for women who live in very dry climates; the moisture that they put out keeps the skin hydrated and makes it more supple-looking. Look for a humidifier that emits only moisture, not warmth.

Loofah

Skin looks best when you exfoliate regularly to slough off dead skin cells. A loofah is a handy product for exfoliating and smoothing the skin on the body; you can use it daily so that your skin always looks fresh and healthy.

Lubriderm Lotion

Lubriderm lotion is fine for most skin types and can be used on the face as well as the body. It hydrates without clogging pores or leaving a greasy film on the skin. An added bonus: It's also available with SPF 15.

Manicure and Pedicure Kits

Your local drugstore is a great place to put together the essentials you need for home manicures and pedicures. I think that Revlon and Sally Hansen give you the best quality for your money.

Maybelline Great Lash Mascara

Maybelline Great Lash Mascara is a longtime favorite of professional makeup artists and other beauty mavens. It's compatible with most eyes, doesn't irritate, stays on all day, and washes off easily at night.

Pantene Pro V Shampoo and Conditioner

Pantene Pro V Shampoo and Conditioner is moisturizing and gentle enough for color-treated hair. And it really does make your hair super-shiny.

Revlon Eyelash Curler

You'd be amazed at what simply curling your eyelashes can do to perk up your eyes. Revlon makes the classic eyelash curler.

Super-Moisturizing Body Creams

Good old cocoa butter is highly moisturizing. Two of my other favorite moisturizers are Nivea Cream and Nivea Body Oil. But these body moisturizers must be used when you have time to let them soak into the skin — try applying them after a relaxing evening bath.

Chapter 18

Ten Terrific Finds at a Beauty Supply Store, Salon, or Specialty Shop

● ●

In This Chapter

▶ Saving money by shopping at a beauty supply

▶ Finding fantastic products at beauty supplies, salons, and specialty shops

● ●

Most women know that salons sell products, but many women don't know — or don't take advantage of — other great resources: beauty supply stores and specialty shops. These stores cater both to professionals and to regular consumers (sometimes the pros pay a bit less) and offer lots of makeup, skin care, and hair care products that you can't find at drugstores. This chapter lists some of the products that I always purchase at a salon, beauty supply, or specialty shop.

Blow-Dryer

If you use a blow-dryer, you're already well aware that a good one can make all the difference in how long it takes to dry your hair and how the end result turns out. It's better to buy a blow-dryer at a beauty supply store because you can normally get a higher wattage than at a drugstore — and the pros say that you should dry hair as quickly as possible. Look for at least 1,500 watts.

Bubble Bath

For bubble bath — which I can't live without — I go to a specialty shop, such as Bath & Body Works, Victoria's Secret, or The Body Shop. Nothing relaxes me more at the end of the day than a hot bath with bubbles that are scented to suit my mood.

Clarifying Shampoo

As Chapter 5 explains, clarifying shampoo is great for removing product build-up and restoring shine and body to the hair. Most hair types benefit from weekly or monthly cleansing with a clarifier. Because it's a "specialized" shampoo, it can be more difficult to find at drugstores, so look for it at your salon, beauty supply store, or specialty shop.

Deep Conditioners and Protein Packs

A deep conditioner or protein pack can perform miracles on chemically damaged (from color or other chemical processing) or very dry hair. Salons and beauty supply stores are great sources of heavy-duty conditioners that *really* moisturize and restore a healthy look to the hair.

Essential Oils for the Bath

Essential oils in a pure form are hard to find. But they're available at many health food stores and specialty shops. Ask the employees for their purest form of essential oil — the purer the oil, the better the effects. My favorites are lavender and tuberose.

Eye Pencils

Eye pencils don't vary much from the least to the most expensive, so you don't necessarily have to splurge on an expensive department store or boutique product, especially if you're not sure of the color or you want to experiment. Beauty supply stores carry a wide variety of eye pencils, and you're usually allowed to test them on your hand.

Hair Brushes

Beauty supply stores generally carry a range of professional brushes — brushes that are great for long hair, brushes that are great for short hair, and everything in between. (Denman and Mason Pearson make terrific basic brushes.) If you opt to purchase your brushes at a salon, the advantage is that your stylist can help you choose the brushes that work best with your particular cut and hair type — especially helpful when you get a new style and need to change your styling methods.

Hairstyling Products

Again, variety is the key here: Beauty supply stores and salons sell *many* different products, and they often have products that take advantage of the latest scientific developments. When you purchase products at a salon, the staff can help you determine which products are best for your hair.

Makeup

Although you can get great makeup at drugstores, the upside to a beauty supply, salon, or specialty shop is that testers are usually available. Colored lip glosses are fun to buy at your local beauty supply, too. Specialty shops like Shu Uemura and M.A.C. are great places to purchase all kinds of makeup if you don't want to do the department store thing.

Makeup Brushes

Whenever I talk about makeup brushes, I emphasize that investing in quality is very important. Although department store brushes are great, they can be quite costly. At a beauty supply, you can still get good quality, but you'll pay less. Another option is to look for high-quality brushes at an artists' supply store.

Perfume

Every woman wants to have her own unique scent. Mixing your own oils, which you can do at many specialty shops, is a unique way to go. Also, most specialty shops have scents that are not as commercial; therefore, you probably won't be wearing the same perfume as your girlfriend. Encounter, a light, fresh scent made by Victoria's Secret, is one of my favorites.

Square- or Round-Tip Tiny Scissors

A pair of tiny scissors is essential for trimming facial or brow hairs that grow too long. Most beauty supply stores carry high-quality scissors at reasonable prices.

Tweezers

Regular drugstore tweezers usually aren't good enough for precision brow shaping; a beauty supply store or specialty shop is a better place to buy them. Look for Tweezerman brand — a perennial favorite of makeup artists and other beauty industry professionals.

Chapter 19

Ten+ Ways to Vary Your Makeup Look

In This Chapter

▶ Simple things you can do to get different effects from your makeup products

▶ Application tips for foundation, blush, mascara, and lip color

*L*ike most women, you may put your makeup on the same way every day because you're rushed. Or maybe you're bored with your look, and next thing you know, you're at the cosmetic counter spending lots of money on products you really don't need. This chapter shows you several ways to vary the look of your foundation, blush, mascara, and lip color without spending a dime.

Foundation

If you've done your homework and found your perfect shades of foundation, powder, and concealer (see Chapter 11 for help with that), you have the three tools you need to give your skin all kinds of great finishes and effects. Varying your look is simply a matter of technique — and the following table tells you how to do it.

To Get This	Do This
"Un-made-up" skin	Use foundation in T-zone only; finish with very little powder or use concealer only, and only where needed; blend well.
Dewy skin	Moisturize entire face before applying foundation; or sheer down foundation with moisturizer or water; and/or dust powder lightly onto forehead, nose, and chin only.

To Get This	Do This
Matte skin	Press loose powder firmly into skin with a puff; whisk off excess with a powder brush or soft baby brush.
Ultra coverage	Apply two layers of foundation; use a puff to press loose powder evenly over skin. Then whisk off loose powder with a powder brush or soft baby brush.

Blush

Bored with your blush shade but can't find one that you like better? Finding a new color may not be the issue — perhaps it's just a question of application innovation. The following table gives you some great options.

To Get This	Do This
Ultra-natural blush	Use cream blush and sheer it down with moisturizer before applying; or use lipstick instead of blush and use little or no powder on cheeks.
Sun-kissed look	Sweep blush over cheeks, chin, forehead, and nose — places the sun naturally hits; or use bronzer instead of blush (see "Working the Extras" in Chapter 14 for more on bronzer).

Mascara

Most women put on mascara exactly the same way every day, but as the following table shows, you can get a lot of different effects from that one little tube. To vary your look even more, try curling your lashes or even just the outer third with a corner curler.

To Get This	Do This
Ultra-natural lashes	Use only a single, thin coat; and/or place color on lash-ends only; and/or comb through lashes while mascara is still wet; and/or hold wand vertically and apply color to lashes one at a time with the tip of the wand.

To Get This	Do This
Very full-looking lashes	Use multiple coats, combing only after applying all coats; and/or use color on both upper- and under-sides of lashes.
Wider-set eyes	Use mascara only on outer third of upper lashes.
Closer-set eyes	Concentrate mascara on the inner two-thirds of lashes.

Lip Color

You have your magic lip-toned pencil and your favorite medium-creamy, medium-coverage lip color. As the following table explains, you can get a variety of lip looks with just those two items.

To Get This	Do This
Ultra-natural lips	Coat lips with lip balm before lightly applying color; and/or apply lipstick to finger and then pat color onto lips; and/or lightly tap on lip color from tube; or lightly line lips with pencil and then top with lip balm to blend line.
Glossy lips	Add a slick of vitamin E, petroleum jelly, or lip balm over lipstick; or coat lips with petroleum jelly and then fill in color with lip pencil.
Ultra-matte lips	Apply color over a base of foundation and blot well; or color in lips completely with lip liner, topping with a little lip balm if lips look too dry.
"Stained" lips	Work lipstick deeply into lips with fingertip; blot until no moisture remains; repeat or color in lips entirely with pencil; rub lip balm lightly into lips with finger; blot down to a stain; and finish with lip balm if lips feel dry.
Lightened color	Give lips a base coat of foundation or concealer or mix foundation or concealer with lip color before applying.

Appendix A
Glossary of 100+ Beauty Terms

Accutane: The prescription drug isotretinoin, used to clear up acne.

acid-balanced perm: A perm that utilizes a gentler chemical and a lower pH than alkaline perms do. Although not as harsh as alkaline perms, acid-balanced perms must be left on longer and activated with heat. They are best for fragile or previously processed hair, or for softer curl effects.

acidic rinse: An after-shampoo rinse with a mildly acidic pH that works to close the cuticle of the hair, improving smoothness and shine. Typical ingredients include vinegar and citrus extracts such as grapefruit and lemon.

acne: A chronic inflammation of the skin's sebaceous (or oil) glands, believed to stem from a few causes: overactive oil glands stimulated by hormonal activity, oversensitivity to even normal levels of hormones, a bacteria, and genetics.

age spot: A concentrated area of pigment that appears on an area of the skin that has endured years of damaging sun exposure.

alkaline: Having a pH higher than 7.

alkaline perm: A perm that uses a strongly alkaline chemical ingredient and tends to give the fastest and longest-lasting results. This type of perm is best for hard-to-curl hair, or for creating a strong or tightly curled effect.

alopecia: Thinning of the hair.

alpha hydroxy acids (AHAs): The generic name for lactic, malic, and glycolic acids that are used in skin care products to exfoliate and moisturize the skin by chemically removing the dead cells from the skin's surface.

antioxidants: These vitamins are often added to foundations and moisturizers and act as free-radical fighters right at the skin's surface. Derivatives of vitamins A, C, and E are the most commonly used antioxidant ingredients.

aromatherapy: Treatments and products that use the scents of herbs, flowers, fruits, and other plants that are known to have therapeutic properties.

ashy: Skin or makeup with gray undertones.

astringent: A skin care product that removes surface skin cells, soap residue, and oils. It usually contains alcohol, which can be drying.

backcomb: To comb the hair back onto itself for the purpose of adding lift, usually done with a teasing comb. Backcombing is also known as teasing.

base: See *foundation*.

benzoyl peroxide: An ingredient used in skin cleansers and other products to dry the skin and clear up blemishes.

beta hydroxy acid (BHA): A derivative of aspirin that's used in skin care products to accelerate skin cell turnover and help clear pores. It penetrates more deeply into the pores than AHAs, so it's effective for anti-acne use.

blackhead: A plug that is open to the air at the skin's surface; exposure to the air is responsible for the dark color.

bleaching cream: A skin-lightening product that's used to even out areas of hyperpigmentation. It works by inhibiting melanin production.

"blue" shampoo: A shampoo that contains blue or violet pigments, made specifically for gray hair.

body wave: A variation on the traditional perm, done with large-diameter rods that create a gentle wave pattern in the hair.

botanicals: Naturally derived oils and aqueous extracts of plants such as rosemary, peppermint, and sage that add a fragrance to a product.

Botox: An injection that temporarily prevents you from making certain facial contractions, such as furrowing your brow, by paralyzing the muscles into which it's injected. The result is a smoother appearance of facial lines and wrinkles.

broad-spectrum: A term used to describe products that have been shown to protect against both UVA and UVB rays.

bronzer: Copper- or gold-toned powder or cream that's used to create a suntanned look.

chemical peel: A procedure that prompts the skin to shed and encourages the growth of fresh, smooth skin. Three types are available: AHA peels, TCA peels, and phenol peels.

clarifying lotion: See *astringent*.

clarifying shampoo: A shampoo that removes product build-up and contains few or no conditioning agents.

cold sore: A red, blistery sore that usually occurs around the mouth and is often accompanied by tingling or discomfort.

collagen: A fiber that's responsible for skin's resilience and flexibility.

collagen injection: A procedure that injects bovine collagen into the skin to plump up wrinkles and depressed scars.

concealer: A heavier, more opaque type of foundation used to cover scars, blemishes, discolorations, and other skin flaws. Comes in liquid, cream, stick, and corrective formulas.

conditioning shampoo: A shampoo that also contains conditioner — a two-in-one product.

contour: To "reshape" the face by using darker shades of blush or foundation to add definition to different features of the face.

contour color: The darkest shade of eye shadow when three shades are used, generally placed in the eye's crease.

cuticle: The hair's outermost layer, which covers and protects the layers beneath. Also, the protective skin at the base of the fingernails and toenails that keeps foreign particles from getting under the skin.

cyst: A small, enclosed deposit of cellular debris and sebum within the skin that shows up as a bump on the skin's surface.

cystic acne: A condition that occurs when a blocked pore ruptures deeply under the skin, causing an infected boil.

dandruff shampoo: A shampoo that contains FDA-regulated ingredients proven to relieve dandruff. It helps control dandruff itching and recurrence.

demipermanent color: A hair color formula that's permanent but that contains less peroxide and dye than fully permanent formulas.

depilatory: A chemical-based lotion or cream that dissolves hair at the skin's surface.

depth: A fancy word for a very basic concept in hair color: light, medium, or dark.

dermabrasion: A procedure that involves sanding the top layer of skin cells from the face or body with a wire brush.

dermatologist: A medical doctor who specializes in treatment of the skin.

dermis: The skin's thicker underlayer, where the skin's sebacious (or oil) glands are located.

detangler: A very lightweight liquid or lotion, sometimes found in spray form, that contains no real conditioning properties but removes tangles and gives hair more manageability and shine.

dewy: Appearing moist — usually used to describe fresh, natural-looking skin.

double-process: Any service where two steps are required to achieve the final look. The classic example of double-processing is going from very dark hair to blonde; first, the majority of color must be stripped from the hair with a bleaching product, and then the final, permanent color is applied (and toned if needed).

dusting: A very slight trim that takes off only the very ends of your hair. Ask for a dusting when you're growing out your hair.

elastin: A fiber that's responsible for skin's resilience and flexibility.

emollient: An oil-based ingredient that is added to hair care and skin care products to retain moisture.

epidermis: The skin's outer layer, where new cells are produced.

essential oil: A pure, concentrated, fragrant oil that's used in aromatherapy.

exfoliate: To remove dead cells from the surface of the skin either chemically with AHA creams or manually with a washcloth or a mildly abrasive product.

fat transplant: A procedure that involves taking fat from a donor site (such as the thighs or buttocks) and injecting it into areas that need plumping — commonly used on facial wrinkles, pitted scars, and lips.

feathering: When lip color falls into the small creases around the mouth, creating a "feathery" look. This can be avoided by using lip liner.

fill: To use color, conditioner, or both together to "fill" porous hair (either in certain areas or all over the head) prior to application of the final color formula. Helps very damaged, overprocessed hair hold color better and get even, uniform results.

finishing rinse: A lightweight, very liquid conditioner formula that detangles and conditions without weighing hair down.

foil: See *highlight*.

gloss: See *demipermanent color*.

glycerin: A humectant that attracts water. It has long been used to hydrate chapped skin, and it's a common ingredient in moisturizers.

hair mask: Similar to a protein pack, but may include clay and/or minerals. Hair masks are good for boosting the health of oily hair because clay draws out moisture.

highlight: To lighten selected strands of hair as opposed to dyeing the entire head. You can highlight with any color that's lighter than what's already there. Strands are often wrapped in foil to keep them separate during processing (which is why highlighting is also known as foiling).

highlight shade: The lightest shade of eye shadow when three are used, usually placed above the eye's crease.

hot oil treatment: A mixture of different oils (plant, animal, or silicone), typically combined with conditioning ingredients like panthenol and proteins, that helps seal in moisture and adds softness to the hair.

humectant: An ingredient added to skin care and hair care products that attracts water to the skin and hair to keep them feeling moisturized.

hyperpigmentation: An overabundance of melanin, which is usually traced to sun exposure, medications (including birth control pills), pregnancy, hormones, and age.

hypopigmentation: The loss of melanin, often due to genetics, skin resurfacing techniques, and just plain aging.

instant conditioner: A conditioner with light to intense conditioning properties that restores a healthy look and protects against further damage.

keloid: A hard, thick, irregularly colored area of skin that results from pronounced overgrowth of tissue. Severe acne and surgery are typical causes.

laser removal: A procedure that corrects pigmentation problems and vascular flaws by emitting a wavelength of light that seeks and pulverizes a certain color in the skin (the color of the problem area).

laser resurfacing: A procedure that works by simultaneously vaporizing the upper levels of the skin and tightening the collagen layer beneath. Gives the skin a smoother appearance.

leave-in conditioner: A conditioner formula with light to medium conditioning properties that is left on the hair, not rinsed out.

level: A fancy word for the broadest possible groupings of hair colors: blonde, red, brown, or black.

lowlight: To weave deeper-toned strands throughout the hair to give color depth and dimension — often used as a repair technique for overlightened hair. Lowlighting is the opposite of highlighting.

mask: A skin care product that's left on the skin for a period of time in order to clean pores and slough off dead cells. Masks come in many formulas, including clay, moisturizing, peel-off and rub-off, and soothing.

matte: Flat-looking rather than shiny or shimmery.

melanin: The substance that determines your natural skin tone and turns skin darker when you tan.

melasma: Also known as "mask of pregnancy," a condition that usually causes darkened skin to appear across the cheek-forehead-nose area.

mica: A finely ground mineral that can flake into eyes and cause redness and irritation, usually found in shimmery eye shadows.

moisturizer: Liquid- or cream-based emollients that provide a lightweight shield that keeps your skin's natural moisture from evaporating — and your skin feeling comfortable.

moisturizing shampoo: A shampoo that contains ingredients that replenish hair's moisture, cleansing without drying.

mole: A little brown bump on the skin. Moles must be watched carefully because they can turn cancerous.

multiphase makeup: Makeup that settles into two distinct parts that you have to shake to mix — typically alcohol or water on top, talc and pigment on the bottom.

oily hair shampoo: A shampoo, formulated specially for oily hair, that dries excess oil at the scalp.

pancake makeup: Also known as stick makeup, a product that's applied alone or over foundation on areas that need extra coverage.

panthenol: A vitamin B$_5$ derivative that is able to penetrate the hair's shaft and add moisture.

perm: To add curl or wave to the hair by using chemicals. Although rods are usually placed horizontally, there are dozens of possible configurations depending on rod size, number of rods, and desired effect.

permanent color: A hair color formula that lasts until the hair is cut off. This type of color covers gray completely.

photoaging: Aging that occurs due to repeated, prolonged exposure to the sun.

polymer: An ingredient used in hairstyling products that coats and separates hairs to create the look and feel of more volume.

protein pack: Similar to a daily conditioner, but with a more intense consistency. It's meant to be left on the hair, sometimes with heat, to allow the hair shaft to open up and absorb moisture.

relax: To chemically straighten the hair to gently smooth out curl, reduce frizz, or create a straight style.

Retin-A: See *tretinoin*.

reverse perm: Actually a method of straightening hair, a technique that uses large-diameter rods to reset tightly curled hair into a looser, more manageable curl pattern.

rinse: See *temporary color*.

root perm: A perm in which rods are placed at the hair's roots only to give lift and volume, or to curl new grow-out when the rest of the hair has been permed previously.

rosacea: A skin problem that resembles acne but is actually a disorder of the blood vessels. It is most common in fair-skinned women over 20 years of age, and is typified by facial ruddiness and red, pimple-like bumps in the cheek and nose areas. Sometimes referred to as acne rosacea or adult acne.

salicylic acid: Also known as BHA. A derivative of aspirin that's used to treat acne and help keep skin clear.

sebaceous glands: The glands of the skin and scalp that produce oil.

sebum: Oil that's produced by the skin and scalp.

semipermanent color: A hair color formula that lasts up to 12 shampoos.

shimmer: A shimmery product that's used to highlight specific areas of the face and body.

silicone: An ingredient used in hairstyling products that smoothes and seals the hair's cuticle so that water can't penetrate it, thereby preventing frizz.

single-process: A color service in which the final look can be achieved by using one formula. Usually refers to permanent color.

SPF: Stands for sun protection factor. The measure of a sunscreen that indicates the product's ability to block out the sun's harmful UVB rays that cause sunburn and skin cancer.

spider vein: A small, red vein that's usually caused by pregnancy, hormonal imbalance, or genetic predisposition.

spiral perm: A perm in which hair is rolled vertically rather than horizontally to create long, corkscrew-type curls.

spot perm: A perm in which perm rods are used only on certain areas of the hair to add body where needed.

straighten: To apply a strong chemical formula (usually sodium hydroxide) to hair, comb the hair as straight as possible, rinse, and neutralize to set the shape.

surfactants: Molecules that dissolve oil-based minerals on the skin.

temporary color: A hair color formula that lasts only until you shampoo your hair.

tester: A sample of a product that you can try out to see whether you like the product and want to buy it.

texturize: To comb relaxer through the hair and leave it in briefly to loosen the curl pattern. The hair is slightly straightened, which makes it look longer and improves manageability.

thickening mascara: A heavier mascara formula that builds up a volumizing coat of color on the lashes.

tinted moisturizer: A moisturizer that contains a bit of color. It's great for everyday use — the color is just enough to even out your skin tone, and it looks like you have no makeup on.

tone: A hair color's underlying shade, which usually falls into one of three categories: warm, cool, or neutral. Also, to use temporary, semi-, or demipermanent color to play up or eliminate tones. In salons, toning is the finishing step for hair that's been lightened dramatically. For example, if hair's too brassy after highlighting, a colorist applies an ash-hued toner to dampen the red.

toner: A skin care product that's used after cleansing and exfoliation to remove any excess oils, freshen the skin, tighten pores temporarily, and return the skin to its natural pH.

translucent powder: Finely ground powder that has less pigment than other pressed or loose powders.

tretinoin: A vitamin A derivative that's used to treat acne. Commonly referred to by its trade name, Retin-A.

trichologist: A professional who analyzes the hair and scalp to determine possible causes of hair problems.

T-zone: The forehead, nose, and chin areas, which tend to be oilier than the cheeks. Breakouts often occur in the T-zone.

undertone: One of the biggest buzzwords in makeup, used to describe the underlying tone of the skin. Most common is a yellowish cast; orange, red, blue, and green are other possibilities. Most foundation formulas are based on those shades.

UVA rays: The sun's aging rays. Sunscreens protect skin against these rays.

UVB rays: The sun's burning rays. Only zinc oxide and titanium dioxide, which are physical sunblocks (they are opaque and coat the skin), are fully able to shield skin from these rays.

vitiligo: The absence of melanin in certain areas of the skin. On the face, the lack of pigment is usually seen around the mouth and eyes.

volumizer: A product that adds fullness to the hair.

volumizing shampoo: A shampoo that contains water-attracting ingredients to swell the hair shaft.

waxing: A method of hair removal that uses hot wax to pull hairs from the follicle.

weave perm: See *spot perm*.

whitehead: A plug of sebum that remains under the skin.

witch hazel: An ingredient used in some toners that combines an extract from the witch hazel shrub with alcohol and water.

Appendix B

Beauty Resources

• •

*I*f you want more information about a particular topic, or you have trouble finding specific beauty-related products, this appendix can help. Here, you'll find listings of organizations, beauty manufacturers, and Web sites. I've also listed the specific makeup shades used to create the looks in the color section of the book for your reference.

Organizations

American Academy of Dermatology
930 N. Meacham Rd.
Schaumburg, IL 60173-6016
847-330-0230
www.aad.org

American Academy of Facial, Plastic, and Reconstructive Surgery
444 E. Algonquin Rd.
Arlington Heights, IL 60005
847-228-9900

American Board of Dermatologists
313-874-1088

American Cancer Society
19 W. 56th St.
New York, NY 10019
212-586-8700
www.cancer.org

American Society for Dermatologic Surgery
930 N. Meacham Rd.
Schaumburg, IL 60173-6016
847-330-0230
www.aad.org

American Society of Plastic and Reconstructive Surgeons
444 E. Algonquin Rd.
Arlington Heights, IL 60005
847-228-9900
www.plasticsurgery.org

Center for Devices and Radiological Health
Food and Drug Administration
5600 Fishers Ln.
Rockville, MD 20857
800-638-2041
www.fda.gov/cdrh

Centers for Disease Control and Prevention
Division of Cancer Prevention and Control
4770 Buford Highway, NE K-64
Atlanta, GA 30341
770-488-4751
www.cdc.gov

Cleveland Clinic Foundation
Department of Dermatology and
Department of Plastic Surgery
9500 Euclid Ave.
Cleveland, OH 44195
800-223-2273

Consumer Federation of America
1424 16th St. NW, Ste. 604
Washington, DC 20036
202-387-6121

Consumer Information Center
P. O. Box 100
Pueblo, CO 81002
888-8-PUEBLO
www.pueblo.gsa.gov

Cosmetic Ingredient Review
1101 L St. NW
Washington, DC 20408
202-331-0651

Cosmetic, Toiletry, and Fragrance
Association
1101 L St. NW
Washington, DC 20408
202-331-1770
www.ctfa.org

Federal Trade Commission
Office of Consumer Education
Bureau of Consumer Protection
Washington, DC 20580
202-326-3650
www.ftc.gov

Food and Drug Administration
Office of Consumer Affairs
5600 Fishers Ln.
Rockville, MD 20857
301-827-4420
www.fda.gov

National Alopecia Areata Foundation
710 C St., Ste. 11
San Rafael, CA 94901
415-456-4644

National Cancer Institute
Department of Health & Human Services
9000 Rockville Pike
Building 31, Room 10A24
Bethesda, MD 20892
800-4-CANCER
www.nci.nih.gov

National Institute of Allergy and
Infectious Diseases
Department of Health & Human
Services
Office of Communications
31 Center Dr.
MSC 2520
Room 7A-50
Bethesda, MD 20892-2520
301-496-5717
www.niad.nih.gov

National Institute of Arthritis and
Musculoskeletal and Skin Diseases
1 AMS Circle
Bethesda, MD 20892-3675
301-495-4484
www.nih.gov/niams

National Institute on Aging
Department of Health & Human
Services
P. O. Box 8057
Gaithersburg, MD 20898-8057
800-222-2225
www.nih.gov/nia

National Rosacea Society
800 S. Northwest Hwy., Ste. 200
Barrington, IL 60010
888-NO-BLUSH
www.rosacea.org

National Vitiligo Foundation
P. O. Box 6337
Tyler, TX 75711
903-531-0074
www.nvfi.org

Office of Cosmetics and Colors
Food and Drug Administration
200 C St. SW
Washington, DC 20204
800-270-8869
www.fda.gov

Skin Cancer Foundation
245 Fifth Ave., Ste. 403
New York, NY 10016
212-725-5176

Manufacturers

Adrien Arpel
888-206-2222
members.aol.com/tjkilmu/adrien/
arpel.html

Alberto-Culver
708-450-3000
www.alberto.com

Alcone
718-361-8373

Aloe Advantage
800-433-5303
In Canada 817-468-3181

Alpha Hydrox/Neoteric
800-55-ALPHA
www.alpha-hydrox.com

Aqua Glycolic
800-253-9499

Aqua Net
800-626-7283

Aussie
www.aussiehair.com

Aveda
800-328-0849
www.aveda.com

Avon
800-FOR-AVON
In Canada 800-265-2866
www.avon.com

Ball Beauty Supply
213-655-2330

Basis
800-227-4703

Bath & Body Works
800-395-1001
www.intimatebrands.com

BeautiControl
800-BEAUTI-1
www.beauticontrol.com

Beauty Without Cruelty
707-769-5120
animals.co.za/Orgs/BWC

BeneFit
800-781-2336

Better Botanicals
888-BBHERBS

Biotherm
888-BIOTHERM

Bobbi Brown Cosmetics
212-980-7040
www.bobbibrowncosmetics.com

The Body Shop
800-541-2535
In Canada 800-387-4592
www.the-body-shop.com

Bonne Bell Cosmetics
800-321-1006
www.bonnebell.com

Breck
800-457-8739

Bumble and Bumble
800-7-BUMBLE
www.bumbleandbumble.com

Cellex-C
800-423-5539

Cetaphil
www.cetaphil.com

Chanel
212-688-5055
www.chanel.com

Chesebrough-Pond's
800-626-7283
In Canada 800-243-5804

Christian Dior
212-759-1840

Clairol
800-223-5800
www.clairol.com

Clarins
212-980-1800

Clean & Clear
800-526-3967

Clearasil
www.clearasil.com

Clinique
212-572-3800
www.clinique.com

C. O. Bigelow Chemists, Inc.
800-793-LIFE

Color Me Beautiful
800-533-5503

Coty
212-850-2300

Cover Girl
888-COVERGIRL
www.covergirl.com

Crabtree & Evelyn
800-272-2873
www.crabtree-evelyn.com

Decleor USA
800-722-2219

Delux Beauty
888-DELUX-BP

Denorex
800-322-3129
In Canada 201-660-5500

Dep Corporation
800-326-2855
In Canada 310-604-0777

DermaBlend
800-621-6043
www.sheen.com/sheen/derma/
dblend.htm

Dermalogica
800-831-5150
www.dermalogica.com

Dermalogics
310-352-4784

Donna Karan Beauty Company
212-572-4200
www.donnakaran.com

Dudley's
800-334-4150

Elizabeth Arden
212-261-1000
www.utee.com/arden

Estee Lauder
212-572-4433

Eucerin
800-227-4703
In Canada 203-853-8008

Excelsior
800-236-6001
In Canada 612-949-3374

Faberge Organics
800-243-5804

FACE Stockholm
888-334-FACE

Fashion Fair
800-631-2158

Finesse
800-621-3379
In Canada 514-457-4111

Focus 21
800-832-2887

Forever Spring
800-523-4334
www.foreverspring.com

Framesi
800-245-6323
In Toronto 416-252-9591
www.framesi.it

Frederic Fekkai Beauté
888-FFEKKAI

Freeman
310-286-0101

Galderma
800-582-8225
www.infoderm.com

Garden Botanika
800-968-7842

Goldwell
800-333-2442
In Canada 800-387-4910

Graham Webb
800-869-9322
In Canada 612-476-4800

Guerlain
800-882-8820
www.guerlain.com

Guinot
800-444-6621
www.lotions.com/guinot

H2O Plus
800-242-BATH

Halsa
800-326-2855
In Canada 310-604-0777

Hard Candy Cosmetics
310-289-7767
www.hardcandy.com

Hayashi
800-448-9500

Head & Shoulders
800-723-9569
In Canada 800-668-0151
www.jnj.com

Helene Curtis
800-621-3379
In Canada 514-457-4111
www.yoursalon.com

Hydron
800-449-3766

Il Makiage
800-722-1011
www.nycbest.com/ilmakiage.htm

Image
800-421-8528

Iman
800-366-IMAN
www.sheen.com/sheen/iman

Infusium
800-223-5800

Jacques Dessange
800-882-8865
www.dessange.com

Jafra
800-551-2345
www.galaxymall.com/retail/
jafra.com

Jane Cosmetics
800-820-JANE
www.janecosmetics.com

Japonesque
800-955-6662

Jheri Redding
800-326-6247
In Canada 604-426-1300
www.conair.com

Jhirmack
800-222-0453
In Canada 201-265-8000

John Frieda
800-521-3189
In Canada 203-762-1233

Johnson&Johnson
800-526-3967
In Canada 800-265-8383
www.jnj.com

Joico
800-44-JOICO
www.joico.com

Kenra
800-428-8073
In Canada317-356-6491

Kiehl's
800-KIEHLS-1

KMS
800-DIALKMS
www.kmshaircare.com

L'anza
800-423-0307
In Canada 818-334-9333

LA Looks
800-326-2855
In Canada 310-604-0777
www.lalooks.com

Lancôme
800-LANCOME
www.loreal.com

Langé
800-227-1406

La Prairie
800-821-5718
www.laprairie.com

Laura Mercier
888-MERCIER

J. F. Lazartigue
800-359-9345

Logics
800-356-4427
In Canada 800-363-0731

Look Good, Feel Better
905-629-0111
www.lgfb.ca

LORAC
800-845-0705

L'Oreal
800-631-7358
In Canada 800-898-2328
www.lorealcosmetics.com

Lori Davis
800-832-4430
In Canada 416-282-1201

Lubriderm
800-223-0182
In Canada 416-288-2200
www.skinhelp.com

Luster's Pink
800-621-4255

M.A.C.
800-387-6707

Make Up For Ever
800-757-5175

Mane 'N' Tail
800-827-9815

Marcelle
800-387-7710

Mary Kay, Inc.
800-MARYKAY
In Canada 905-858-2026
www.marykay.com

Mastey
800-6-MASTEY

Matrix
800-6-MATRIX
In Canada 800-833-2861
www.matrix-cosmetics.nl

Max Factor
800-526-8787

Maybelline
800-944-0730
www.loreal.com

M. D. Formulations
800-253-9499
In Canada 800-738-3223

Merle Norman Studios
800-40-MERLE

Molton Brown Cosmetics
800-787-2550

Mon Amie
800-983-3000

Murad
800-59-MURAD
In Canada 310-568-1940

Nailtiques
800-272-0054

Naomi Sims Beauty Center
800-556-SIMS

Nars
888-903-NARS

NeoStrata
800-628-9904
In Canada 215-624-4224
www.neostrata.com

Neutrogena
800-421-6857
310-642-1150
www.neutrogena.com

Nexxus
800-444-6399
In Canada 805-968-6900
www.nexxushair.com

Nioxin
800-628-9890

Nivea
800-233-2340
In Canada 203-853-8008
www.nivea.com

Noevir
800-USA-8888
In Canada 800-465-4655
www.noevirusa.com

Nordstrom Beauty Hotline
800-7-BEAUTY

Norma Kamali Beauty
800-4-KAMALI
www.omo-norma-kamali.com

Nucleic-A
800-444-0699
In Canada 612-571-1234

Nu Skin
801-345-1000
www.nuskin.net

Oil of Olay
800-285-5170
In Canada 800-668-0151

OPI
800-341-9999

Origins
800-ORIGINS

Orlane
800-775-2541

Pantene
800-723-9569
In Canada 800-668-0151

Paul Mitchell
800-793-8790

Pert
800-723-9569
In Canada 800-668-0151

Philosophy
888-2-NEW-AGE
www.philosophy.com

Physicians Formula
800-227-0333

Phytology
800-55-PHYTO

Phytotherathrie
800-648-0349
In Canada 800-363-1660

Ponds Institute
800-34-PONDS
www.ponds-institute.com.my/
main.html

Poppy
212-598-4400

Prescriptives
212-572-4400, ext. 4811
212-756-4801

Princess Marcella Borghese
212-551-7900

Principal Secret
800-545-5595

Pro Active
800-888-8200

Procter & Gamble
800-723-9569
In Canada 800-668-0151
www.pg.com

Purpose
800-526-3967
In Canada 800-265-8383

Quantum
800-621-3379

Rachel Perry
800-966-8888
www.rachelperry.net

Rave
800-626-RAVE
In Canada 800-243-5804

Ray Beauty Supply
212-757-0175

Redken
800-423-5369
212-249-0633
In Canada 212-818-1500

Redmond
800-328-0159
In Canada 905-602-1965

Revlon
800-4-REVLON
In Canada 919-603-2000
www.revlon.com

Ricky's Beauty Supply
212-979-5232

Rusk
800-USERUSK

St. Ives
800-333-6666
In Canada 818-709-5500
www.stives.com

Sally Beauty Supply
800-284-SALLY
www.sallybeauty.com

Salon Selectives
800-621-3379
In Canada 514-457-4111
www.yoursalon.com

Salon Style
800-444-0699
In Canada 612-571-1234

Scarlett Cosmetics
215-862-9408
www.scarlettcos.com

Schwarzkopf
416-441-9933

Scruples
800-457-0016
In Canada 612-469-4646

Sebastian International
800-829-7322

Selsun Blue
800-227-5767
In Canada 800-361-7852

Senscience
800-242-9283
In Canada 800-626-3684

Sephora
212-625-1309

Shiseido
800-354-2160
www.shiseido.co.jp/e/

Shu Uemura
800-743-8205

Soft Sheen
800-621-6143

Sorbie
800-322-8738
In Canada 905-825-5800

Spa Thira
800-76-THIRA
www.spathira.com

Stila
800-883-0400

Style
800-444-0699
In Canada 612-571-1234

Suave
800-621-3379

TIGI
800-256-9391
In Canada 972-931-1567

Tresemme
708-450-3000
www.alberto.com

Tressa
800-879-8737

Tri
800-458-8874

Trish McEvoy
800-431-4306
212-758-7790

Trucco
800-829-7322

Tweezerman
800-645-3340
www.tweezerman.com

Ultima II
800-4-REVLON
In Canada 919-603-2000

Ultra Swim
800-745-2429
In Canada 800-268-3949

Urban Decay
800-784-8722
www.urbandecay.com

Valerie
800-282-5374

Vaseline Intensive Care
800-743-8640

Vibrance
800-621-3379

Victoria Jackson
800-V-MAKEUP
www.vmakeup.com

Victoria's Secret
800-888-8200

Vidal Sassoon
800-262-1637
In Canada 800-668-0151
www.vidalsassoon.co.uk

Wella
800-843-2656
In Canada 800-565-2588

White Rain/Tame
800-872-7202

Yves Rocher
800-321-9837
www.yvesrocherusa.com

Yves St. Laurent
212-246-9494

Zotos
800-242-9283
In Canada 800-626-3684

Beauty-Related Web Sites

www.beautynet.com: The information on this site is composed of contributions from professionals at top salons. Each week, a salon professional reviews a featured product or technique. This site bills itself as a virtual salon, and indeed it has category-specific chat rooms in which the pros offer interactive advice: Post your question and a pro will respond online with suggestions (other readers respond sometimes as well). Additionally, a four-category FAQ section deals with hair, skin care, tanning, and nails. This is a well-put-together site.

www.cologneguy.com: Answers from the Cologne Guy is a great site. The Cologne Guy reviews fragrances, provides a fragrance FAQ section, and gives lots of insider info. He has a straightforward style of explanation, covering basic terms and offering links to other fragrance sites.

www.cosmeticmall.com: Cosmetic Mall is a commercial site that contains some great information. There's a dictionary of cosmetic ingredients (in case you want to find out what cetearyl alcohol is for) and also a Women's Resource Directory — a listing of interesting links to a variety of women's sites. A beauty FAQ section covers basic makeup application.

www.hairnet.com: Hair Net is basically a site for hair industry professionals, but it has sections specifically for consumers as well, providing for the general public an interesting, "backstage" view of the hairstyling industry. Hair Net Hotline is an open exchange of advice, ideas, and opinions covering everything from specific questions about hair problems to commentary on the hairstyles of the Weather Channel's meteorologists. One section is devoted to showing a model with one haircut styled into three or four different looks. There's also a nationwide listing of hair salons.

www.homearts.com - World of Style section: This site offers a compilation of material from several Hearst magazines: *Marie Claire, Redbook,* and *HomeArts.* Handy features include *Redbook*'s Red Alert Makeover (answer questions about your physical characteristics and get four pages of analysis and advice); tips for accenting your beauty from professional hairdressers and makeup artists; and a listing of links to fashion and culture Web sites.

www.kleinman.com - Cosmetic Connection section: This is a four-star site for practical users of makeup. It offers an astonishing range of reviews from real-sounding women on makeup, hair, and skin care products, sorted by makeup line. All the major lines are covered, and many minor ones as well. For some products, more than one review is provided, which gives an interesting perspective. Through the site, you can subscribe to the free weekly electronic newsletter, *The Cosmetic Report.* A makeup artist is on the site to respond to your cosmetic questions.

www.phys.com: This site, titled Nutrition for Normal People, is based on information from *Allure, Glamour,* and *Vogue.* It emphasizes health and wellness, in addition to topics on cosmetics, hair, and so on. Particularly cool are the calculators provided to help you determine your current body fat percentage, Body Mass Index, ideal calorie and fat needs, and so on. A wide variety of nutrition topics are covered, with weekly features and self-quizzes. Also included is an encyclopedia of nutrients and additives, which can tell you what all those big words on food packaging mean.

www.stylexperts.com: Style Experts is run by the big guns: interactive advice on a whole gamut of style, fashion, hair, and skin care topics from the Fashion Famous such as Vera Wang, Nikki Taylor, and Todd Oldham. Particularly cool: Iman on ethnic makeup, Brad Johns on hair color, Laura Mercier on makeup, and Serge Normant on hairstyle. These pros respond online to questions that visitors post to the site. Also provided are links to other beauty and style sites.

www.womenslink.com - Beauty Central section: Sponsored by Bristol-Meyers Squibb, this site provides information about some of the company's beauty-related products (for example, Clairol) but also brings in celebrity consultants for (nonpartisan) technique information about clothing, makeup, and hair. *Entertainment Tonight's* Dorothy Cline-Metz has a section called The Fitting Room, where you can learn how to define your body type in order to choose clothing styles that work to your advantage. Roxanna Floyd, a celebrity makeup artist, provides makeup advice for African-American women. Mimi Vodnoy, another Hollywood type, offers help with hair.

E-Magazines

www.fashionstance.com: Fashion Stance is a free monthly e-magazine that covers topics such as cosmetics, fragrances, and skin care.

www.tlhs.org: The Long Hair Site is a (unintentionally) wacky e-magazine devoted to long hair in all its glory. It includes tips from site visitors on treatment of long hair, information about handling long hair on a seasonal basis, and links to other beauty-related sites.

Also interesting in the world of technology/cosmetics is *Cosmopolitan's* "virtual makeover" CD-ROM, which is supposed to be a very good program.

Makeup Shades Used in the Color Section of This Book

All the makeup used in the color Makeup Workbook is from NARS (for more information about retail outlets near you, call 888-903-NARS). In case you want to duplicate one of the looks for yourself, the following list includes the specific products and shades worn by each model:

Stephanie Seymour, Natural Glamour, pages 2 and 3: Vanilla Concealer, Jodhpur Eyebrow Pencil, All About Eve Duo Eyeshadow (lighter shade), Bengali Single Eyeshadow (used in crease), Black Moon Eyeliner Pencil, Black Orchid Mascara, Flesh Loose Powder, Desire Blush, Salsa Lipliner Pencil, Sunset Strip Lip Gloss

Margaret Seymour, Night & Day, pages 4 and 5:

Natural Day Makeup: Honey Concealer, Malibu Multiple (multi-purpose makeup stick), Bengali Single Eyeshadow (used as brow color), All About Eve Duo Eyeshadow, Bamboo Mascara, Eden Loose Powder

From Day to Evening: Kiki Single Eyeshadow (used wet as liner), Arizona Single Eyeshadow (used in crease), Black Orchid Mascara, Amour Blush, Eden Loose Powder, Belle de Jour Sheer Lipstick, Classified Lip Gloss

Daniela Pestova, Refined Glamour, pages 6 and 7: Ginger Concealer, Santa Fe Foundation, The Multiple (multi-purpose makeup stick, used as blush) in South Beach, Bali Single Eyeshadow (used as brow color), Black Moon Eyeliner Pencil, Sophia Single Eyeshadow (used to blend pencil), Tiger Lily Duo Eyeshadow (lighter shade used all over lid, darker shade used in crease), Black Orchid Mascara, Eden Loose Powder, Viva Las Vegas Sheer Lipstick

Carmen, Timeless Beauty, pages 8 and 9: Honey Concealer, Santa Fe Foundation, The Multiple (multi-purpose makeup stick, used as blush) in Malibu, Madrague Duo Eyeshadow (lighter shade applied wet all over lid, darker shade used dry in crease), Panama Eyebrow Pencil, Bali Single Eyeshadow (used to blend brow pencil), Black Forest Single Eyeshadow (used as eyeliner), Black Orchid Mascara, Beach Loose Powder, Fantasia Lipliner Pencil, Blonde Venus Satin Lipstick

Raquel, Simply Great Skin, page 10: The Multiple (multi-purpose makeup stick) in Waikiki (bronze) and Ibiza (gold shimmer)

Margareth, Beautifully Balanced, pages 10 and 11: Chocolate Concealer, Jamaica and Hawaii Foundation, The Multiple (multi-purpose makeup stick) in Waikiki, Black Moon Eyeliner Pencil (used on brows and eyes), Black Forest Single Eyeshadow, Mountain Loose Powder, Times Square Semi Matte Lipstick

Tatjana, Soft Smokiness, page 12 and 13: Ginger Concealer, Bombshell (pearl gray), Black Forest (black), and Kiki (charcoal gray) Single Eyeshadows, Zen Blush, Bambi Satin Lipstick

Yamila, Strong Smoulder, page 13: Ginger Concealer, Beach Pressed Powder, Blue Lotus and Black Moon Eyeliner Pencils, Arizona and California Single Eyeshadows, Black Orchid Mascara, Rain Lip Therapy

Ling, Focus on Lips, page 14: Vanilla Concealer, Deauville Foundation, Black Moon Eyeliner Pencil, Himalayas Single Eyeshadow, Black Orchid Mascara, Mata Hari Blush, Jungle Red Lipliner Pencil, Jungle Red Semi Matte Lipstick

Index

(continued)

(continued)

(continued)

(continued)

• *W* •

Notes

Notes